Penguin Education

Penguin Science of Behaviour
General Editor: B. M. Foss

Abnormal Psychology
Editor: Max Hamilton

Brain Damage and the Mind
Moyra Williams

Moyra Williams

Brain Damage and the Mind

Penguin Books

Penguin Education,
A Division of Penguin Books Ltd,
Harmondsworth, Middlesex, England
Penguin Books Inc., 7110 Ambassador Road,
Baltimore, Md 21207, U.S.A.
Penguin Books Australia Ltd,
Ringwood, Victoria, Australia

First published 1970
Reprinted 1973
Copyright © Moyra Williams, 1970

Made and printed in Great Britain by
Hazell Watson & Viney Ltd
Aylesbury, Bucks
Set in Monotype Times

Penguin Science of Behaviour

This book is one in an ambitious project, the *Penguin Science of Behaviour*, which covers a very wide range of psychological inquiry. Many of the short 'unit' texts are on central teaching topics, while others deal with present theoretical and empirical work which the Editors consider to be important new contributions to psychology. We have kept in mind both the teaching divisions of psychology and also the needs of psychologists at work. For readers working with children, for example, some of the units in the field of Developmental Psychology deal with psychological techniques in testing children, other units deal with work on cognitive growth. For academic psychologists, there are units in well-established areas such as Learning and Perception, but also units which do not fall neatly under any one heading, or which are thought of as 'applied', but which nevertheless are highly relevant to psychology as a whole.

The project is published in short units for two main reasons. Firstly, a large range of short texts at inexpensive prices gives the teacher a flexibility in planning his course and recommending texts for it. Secondly, the pace at which important new work is published requires the project to be adaptable. Our plan allows a unit to be revised or a fresh unit to be added with maximum speed and minimal cost to the reader.

Above all, for students, the different viewpoints of many authors, sometimes overlapping, sometimes in contradiction, and the range of topics Editors have selected, will reveal the complexity and diversity which exist beyond the necessarily conventional headings of an introductory course.

B.M.F.

Contents

Editorial Foreword 9

Introduction 11

1 Consciousness and Mood 15

2 Disorders of Memory 33

3 Disorders of Perception 58

4 Disorders of Motor Skill and Verbal Expression 93

5 Disorders of General Intelligence and Personality 124

References 156

Index 169

Editorial Foreword

The old style textbook of psychology always had a chapter on the brain and its structure, but this was merely a hat-raising gesture to the principle that the subject matter of psychology is one aspect of the function of the brain. The information provided bore no relation to anything in the rest of the text, and no student would have been inconvenienced in any way had the book-binder accidentally omitted that chapter. Even the texts on physiological psychology were largely concerned with the special senses and the structure of the sense organs. The situation is very different now: there are few areas of psychology, perhaps excluding social psychology, which do not show some influence of our increasing understanding of the higher functions of the brain.

This short book is not concerned with the cerebral basis of behaviour, but with the effects of damage to the brain. There are two ways of looking at the subject: from the viewpoint of functional disturbance and its relation to cerebral damage or the other way round, damage to the brain and its consequences. The latter viewpoint will be represented in another volume. This work has been written from the author's particular viewpoint, concentrating on those aspects of the subject which interest her particularly and to which she has contributed in no small measure by her researches. The reader who studies this book carefully will meet not only a coherent, individual viewpoint, but also sound judgement based on experimental work and clinical experience, expressed with clarity and precision. The student and research worker, the psychologist, neurologist and psychiatrist will all be indebted to Dr Moyra Williams for this book. I am also indebted to her for her willingness to meet the requirements of the Abnormal Psychology section in the Penguin Science of Behaviour series.

M.H

Introduction

It has long been recognized that mental functions which cannot be studied selectively under laboratory conditions in the healthy individual may break down in a circumscribed manner as a result of brain injury or disease. Nature herself performs the experiment and its consequences are open to scientific scrutiny. The study of mental disorders as they are manifested in the clinical setting can, therefore, provide valuable information about the working of the healthy mind, and it is the purpose of this volume to summarize the information gained to date from such studies and analyse the conclusions which may be drawn from them. In addition, neuropsychology – as it has come to be called – has practical value for psychologists, especially those working in the clinical field. Since circumscribed cerebral lesions often cause specific and clearly definable mental dysfunctions, recognition of the latter may provide valuable clues about the presence and location of intracerebral pathology. Furthermore, a close analysis of the methods used by some individuals to overcome, adapt to or compensate for, particular functional disturbances could be of value when planning rehabilitation programmes.

During recent years the work done in this field has been enormous. Some selection has, therefore, had to be made and has been based on three principles. In the first place, the work reported here is almost exclusively confined to that dealing with the human being. For obvious reasons this means observation in the clinical setting. Animal experiments, important though they are, have been mentioned only if directly relevant to clinical observations. But even in the clinical field, the manipulation of factors is possible, allowing for some control over the variables being studied; and evidence from experimental neuropsychology forms a large section of this work.

In the second place, mental activity is considered only in relation to the gross anatomical areas of the brain involved. The effects of variation in the biochemical and electrophysiological activity of this complicated organ are only referred to briefly. Again, this is not because such factors are considered unimportant: on the contrary, they are of such vital import-that whole books have been devoted to them alone.

In the third place, the literature covered here has been restricted almost entirely to that published in the English language. Further selection of this vast bulk of literature has again been necessary and most of the work referred to will be that with which the author has some personal connexion and hence some basis on which to form a judgement.

Even with the above restrictions the amount of data available on the subject of psychological disorders and brain lesions is vast. How to present it most clearly and systematically has been a problem. The material has, in fact, been pressed into five main categories dealing with disorders of (a) Consciousness and Mood, (b) Memory, (c) Perception, (d) Motor Activity, (e) Intelligence and Personality. It cannot be stressed too strongly that there is a great deal of overlap between these categories and they are distinguished by name only. The distinction is based, however, not only on the nature of the functions themselves but also, as will become apparent in the text, on the finding that similar anatomical areas are involved when disorders are seen in each one.

Each section opens with a description of clinical observations and continues with some of the experimental investigations that have been based on them. Finally, the cerebral areas involved in their disturbances have been discussed.

I would like to express my gratitude to those who have made this book possible by encouraging and allowing me to work in this field, particularly Professor W. Ritchie Russell and the late Professor Sir Hugh Cairns who first enticed me into the field of work; to Professors O. L. Zangwill and R. C. Oldfield, pioneers of neuropsychology in this country and still two of its most active and stimulating workers; to Dr L. Z. Cosin for the opportunity to work in geriatrics; and, finally, to the consultants of Littlemore Hospital, Oxford, and Addenbrooke's and Fulbourn Hospitals, Cambridge.

I would like also to thank Dr R. T. Wilkinson and Professor O. L. Zangwill for their comments on the first draft of the present volume; and Professor Karl Pribram, Dr Grey Walter and Dr Elizabeth Warrington for allowing me to read and quote from papers of theirs which are difficult to obtain in this country.

1 Consciousness and Mood

Consciousness and Wakefulness

Responsiveness to outside events is not the prerogative of man or even of animals. Plants respond to light and to the proximity of other plants, while even stones may break up in frost and rain. Where consciousness begins and ends is a philosophical question, but in the clinical field argument is overcome by a strict adherence to the measurement of behaviour. Consciousness is defined by the clinician in terms of the changes in behaviour which follow sensory stimulation, and in this sense it is closely connected, in mammals, with activity within the brain.

Clinical consciousness is by no means an all-or-none phenomenon. Behaviour of different degrees and complexity is seen in different conditions, and in this chapter an attempt will be made to examine the relationship between the level of consciousness observed and the activity of specific areas within the brain.

The levels of consciousness defined in clinical terms are: (a) simple reflex activity; (b) restless and purposeless movements; (c) purposeful movements but no speech or understanding of speech; (d) restless movements and the ability to utter a few words or phrases, often explosive; (e) uninhibited speech and action but disorientation and amnesia for current events; and (f) full orientation and social decorum (Russell, 1959, p. 51).

These levels tend to shade into one another and the transition from one to the next is often difficult to define. Thus, describing one patient suffering from tuberculous meningitis, Williams and Smith (1954) report:

For the first week in hospital he remained drowsy, confused and unable to feed himself. During the second week the acute confusional state lightened. He began to sit up in bed and gradually learnt to feed himself until by the end of twelve days he was alert, friendly and co-operative, but with a gross amnesia for all recent events. Thus he could never remember having seen the ward sister before in spite of the devoted care she gave him. When the trolley was brought for his daily lumbar puncture he would obediently roll over on his side, but as soon as the needle was withdrawn he would deny that he had ever had anything done to his back. He was fully awake all day and occupied himself with handwork or reading the comic strips in the papers, but the moment he was distracted from his occupation, he would have no recollection of what he had been doing the moment before.

Although during the return of consciousness, orientation for person, place and time usually recovers before the ability to retain recent experiences (memory), this is not always the case. Patients often describe 'waking up and not knowing who or where I was', indicating that they have retained a recollection of the situation they were in before regaining all other past memories.

Unconsciousness is differentiated from unwakefulness in that in the former condition the patient can never be fully aroused by external stimuli whereas in the latter he can. There are a number of clinical conditions in which wakefulness rather than consciousness is impaired, a patient tending to fall asleep or to drowse in abnormal circumstances (narcolepsy).

The connexion between the levels of behaviour mentioned above and activity of the brain can be followed on the electro-encephalogram – EEG. This records the electrical activity of the brain by means of electrodes placed on the surface of the skull. These records may mean little to the inexperienced but in the hands of the expert different wave forms can be identified which are found to correspond with different degrees of both consciousness and wakefulness.

Since clinical consciousness may be impaired by a variety of different causes, and since these often result in different clinical pictures, instances and examples of impairments arising from different causes are cited below.

Impairment of consciousness after head injury

In concussional head injury the patient is rendered unconscious immediately, but from then on his degree of responsiveness tends to increase although there may be day-to-day variation. A typical case may be quoted as follows:

A housewife, aged forty-four, who had two children aged ten and eight was knocked off her bicycle on 2.3.51. On admission to hospital she was responding to painful stimuli only but the following day her conscious level deteriorated and her temperature and blood pressure rose. 7.3.51: conscious level began to improve. She would open her eyes and mumble when spoken to but did not obey commands. 15.3.51: it was possible to recognize her mumblings as attempts to form such words as 'all right', 'I don't know'. She could count one and two fingers, but there was much perseveration – i.e. the repetition of one response to succeeding stimuli.

During the following two to three weeks she showed gradual mental improvement and became continent. She appeared to be slightly euphoric. Investigations were carried out which showed very slight dilation of the ventricles inside the brain, but nothing else. For the next five weeks she would talk readily but remained very confused and amnesic. Six weeks after injury there were signs of improvement in memorizing.

9.5.51: nine weeks after injury, she was able to date her accident correctly and believed that she had 'sorted out' most of the misplaced events in her remote past.

29.8.51: she had returned home and was able to lead a full social and domestic life although she still had a number of gaps in her memory for events which had occurred before her injury (Williams, 1954).

Loss of consciousness (and the accompanying amnesia) occur only rarely in head injuries which are not caused by sudden violent changes of direction. Penetrating wounds of the head, even though they may cause severe cortical damage, seldom cause immediate unconsciousness or concussion (Russell, 1959, p. 75).

Impairment of consciousness from intracranial tumours (ICT)

In the case of ICTs the level of consciousness may fluctuate dramatically from moment to moment, the degree of responsiveness present at any one time depending mainly on the area of the brain affected. This point has been demonstrated very clearly by Cairns (1952) who underlines the difference between the levels of consciousness shown by patients with lesions in different parts of the brain and the physiological disorders accompanying them. Thus lesions in the lower brain-stem may

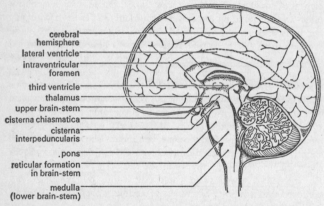

cerebral hemisphere
lateral ventricle
intraventricular foramen
third ventricle
thalamus
upper brain-stem
cisterna chiasmatica
cisterna interpeduncularis
.pons
reticular formation in brain-stem
medulla (lower brain-stem)

Figure 1 Longitudinal section through brain and brain-stem

cause sudden, short intermittent attacks of deep unconsciousness, usually followed quickly by alterations of breathing, irregular pulse, fluctuations of blood pressure and increased tonus of the limbs which together frequently result in death. Lesions in the upper brain-stem and around the thalamus, on the other hand, cause a state more like that of sleep (see Figure 1). Sometimes these too are short and may be accompanied by epileptic fits, the patient remaining fully awake between them and showing no disorders of mentality.

Dramatic examples are quoted by Cairns of patients with cystic tumours in and around the third ventricle, whose level

of consciousness alternated as the cyst filled or was surgically
emptied. When the cyst was full of fluid and causing local
pressure on the floor of the third ventricle, one girl of fourteen

lay inert, except that her eyes followed the movements of objects or
could be diverted by sound. As one approached her bedside her
steady gaze seemed to promise speech, but no sound could be
obtained from her by any form of stimulus. A painful stimulus
would produce reflex withdrawal of the limb and, if the stimulus was
maintained, slow feeble ineffective movements of a voluntary kind
to remove the source of stimulation; but without tears, noise or
other signs of pain or displeasure. She swallowed readily, but had
to be fed; hard food would be swallowed whole, and she would take
sugar, salt or quinine in her mouth without any sign of pleasure or
distaste. There were also mild signs of bilateral pyramidal tract
involvement, and she was totally incontinent.

This patient's third ventricle cyst was aspirated without anaesthe-
sia on several occasions. A needle was passed into the lateral ventricle, where the pressure of cerebrospinal fluid was found to be
normal or nearly normal, and was then advanced into the region of
the third ventricle. Cystic fluid in amounts of 12 to 18 ml was
removed. On one occasion 5 ml of air were then injected to determine the site and extent of the cyst, which occupied the situation of
the third ventricle.

On the first occasion, immediately the cyst was tapped the child
roused and made the first loud sound we had heard from her, but
she would not speak. However, within ten minutes she gave her
name, age and address correctly, without any disorder of articulation, and then asked where she was.

Attacks of hypersomnia, akinetic mutism (the condition
described above in which the patient lies with eyes open
appearing to follow moving objects but making no other
response) and *petit mal* may also occur in lesions around this
area, which Cairns, by a process of deduction based on careful
clinical records, claims must be due to direct involvement of
the area affected by the lesion and cannot be due to generalized
cerebral impairment either from anoxia (due to restricted
bloodflow) or to increased intracranial pressure.

Impairment of consciousness from toxic infective disorders

That consciousness may be disordered from toxic and infective states has long been known. The mental confusion that accompanies any high fever is described in most psychiatric textbooks, and is characterized not so much by loss of responsiveness as by the inappropriateness of the responses made. The patient is disorientated, misinterprets his sensory environment or sees things that are not there (hallucinates), and becomes unable to keep track of time. Of special interest, however, are the disorders which have both a specific effect on discrete cerebral areas and cause selective impairments of consciousness and wakefulness. Of these, encephalitis lethargica and tuberculous meningitis are the best known. Describing the condition of patients in the acute stages of encephalitis lethargica, Mayer Gross, Slater and Roth (1960) point out that disorders of sleep rhythm and mental changes are the most common characteristics. There is

irresistible somnolence which continues for days or weeks. The patient can be aroused to have his meals and often carry on a rational conversation, and if stimulation is maintained he can be kept awake for periods of half to one hour, but left to himself, lethargy soon overpowers him. During sleep there is a marked restlessness and myoclonic jerking. More rarely there is total sleeplessness and inversion of the sleep-rhythm (p. 415).

Accompanying these in the acute phase of the illness may be delirium

marked by vivid, terrifying hallucinations . . . states of delirium may alternate with periods of somnolence, the combination rather characteristic of encephalitis lethargica. Acute stupor is not uncommon and may take a typically catatonic form with negativism and flexibilitas cerea (the tendency to hold the limbs in any position in which they are placed) . . . more universal is a curious affective change . . . marked by emotional immobility with poverty of affective response to all stimuli even when the patient is at his most alert; the death of a wife, a child or a friend is passed by without comment or apparent reaction (p. 416).

In tuberculous meningitis (TBM), an illness which has been recognized for much longer than encephalitis lethargica, Williams and Smith (1954) quote Whytt as noting in 1768 that in the early stages in children, 'their spirits being low they incline mostly to lie in bed, although they are more often disposed to watching than sleep.' This state usually gives way after a short time to an 'amnesic' state which may persist for many months (see chapter 2), during which patients are often rather euphoric but sufficiently alert and rational to occupy themselves and cope adequately (though not yet quite normally) with intellectual problems, but have difficulty in retaining any new impression for more than a few minutes. More will be said about this stage in the following chapter, but here it may be noted in passing that, in TBM as in encephalitis lethargica, the brunt of the disease falls on the base of the brain and particularly on the more anterior of the basal cisterns, the cisternae chiasmaticae and the cisternae interpenduculares (see Figure 1, p. 18).

The mental state in tuberculous meningitis and encephalitis lethargica is distinguished from that seen in other toxic illnesses involving the brain by affecting wakefulness and memory more severely than perception, sensation, and intellectual functions.

Epilepsy

Epileptic seizures are among the commonest causes of disordered consciousness, though not all seizures are followed or accompanied by loss of consciousness. If abnormal electrical activity remains confined to small portions of the cerebrum, it is followed by localized muscular twitching. Only if it becomes generalized to the whole brain does loss of consciousness follow. Epilepsy can thus be classified into partial (or focal) and generalized (Freidman and Kaplan, 1967). Epilepsy can be caused by a great many factors including metabolic disorders (including drug and alcohol withdrawal), cerebrovascular disorders and focal areas of abnormality (due to intracranial tumours, abscesses and cerebral injury) (Ervin, 1967). It can also be caused by abnormally intense sensory stimulation. Thus in those people who have a low threshold to fits frequent rhythmical flashes of light (stroboscope) are a common stimulant: loud noises may fire off fits in a number of people, and even some words (written or spoken) may be sufficient in certain sensitive individuals (Sherwin, 1966). At the same time the onset of a fit may be checked in some subjects by mental effort or by conditioning (see Ervin, 1967). In many cases, however, the causes may never be discovered.

Disorders of consciousness may precede the actual fit, accompany it, follow it, or show themselves as general disorders of personality pervading the patient's whole life.

Sleep

Although all the instances of disordered consciousness described above occur under conditions of cerebral dysfunction, periodic loss of consciousness in sleep is essential to normal waking behaviour.

The differences between sleep and loss of consciousness in coma are, however, considerable. During normal sleep, the sensory system is continually monitoring incoming data, rejecting the insignificant and picking out the significant or rare, in response to which the subject makes appropriate actions and even, if necessary, awakes (e.g. the mother wakes when she hears her child cry; the man used to traffic wakes when it ceases). In between the two extremes of rejection and selection, there is a phase wherein sensory data or preoccupations are woven into a strange half-world of experience called dreams.

In coma, as already described, only intense stimulation is responded to and that usually by little more than reflex movements of the limbs. Moreover the stimuli and the responses which they elicit are not retained as memories.

Over-arousal

Up until now, all impairments of consciousness have been considered in relation to the number and range of environmental events to which the subject does *not* respond. But obviously there are a great many events occurring in our environment the whole time to which responses would be inappropriate and might even reduce efficiency. Consciousness seems to include some mechanism by means of which these stimuli are 'filtered out' before we ever become aware of them. When listening to a conversation in a noisy room, we reject all sounds except those made by the speakers to whom we are attending. We do not notice the daisies growing in a field until we start looking for a golf ball among them. These phenomena will be discussed more fully later on, but in the meantime it may be noted that there are some clinical conditions in which the filtering mechanisms described above seem to go wrong or fail to work. Over-arousal as this reaction is usually called seems to be a basic condition in some psychotic states (McGhie, Chapman and Lawson, 1965) and is often accompanied by abnormal EEG reactions to external stimuli (Hutt *et al.*, 1964).

Psychological factors in altered consciousness

During states of altered or lowered consciousness a number of behavioural characteristics have been indentified.

Loss of vigilance. As might be expected vigilance is lowered. If a subject is placed in a situation in which he has to watch out for intermittent signals, he begins missing some out. This can be of great importance in military and industrial concerns, where a lapse on the part of a fatigued night-watchman might cause the loss of a country or of a million-pound machine. The connexion between vigilance and wakefulness has therefore been studied in detail, and a number of correlated variables has been established. For example, in order for the fatigued subject not to miss signals, he needs longer between the signals to make his responses. The signals have to be greater in intensity in relation to the background noise, and a preliminary alerting signal often helps. Incentive is also of importance. The physiological mechanisms which may explain these findings will be discussed later.

Altered thinking and imagery. As has been described, mental activity becomes altered in character. However, in illnesses which affect mainly wakefulness, the roused patient may still be capable of logical thinking. He can carry out learned behaviour patterns (e.g. use language) appropriately. He can work out quite complex perceptual problems (e.g. play a game of draughts). Moreover, after recovery of the condition causing impaired consciousness, even if this has lasted for many months, intellectual ability seems to return to its previous level. Thus, patients who remained 'unconscious' after head injury, cerebral tumours and tuberculous meningitis for weeks on end have been shown to be capable of resuming their previous occupations or passing intellectual tests at the same high level as before.

Loss of memory retention. The connexion between lowered levels of consciousness and inability to retain impressions is a consistent finding in all clinical material. After concussional head injuries (as opposed to penetrating ones that do not cause loss of consciousness) memory is always to some extent impaired. After illnesses affecting wakefulness, the same phenomenon is seen. Even during sleep, there is a very strong tendency to 'forget' dreams almost immediately after they have occurred. The connexion between consciousness and memory will be considered further in chapter 2.

Disorders of mood. These are again a most common finding in clinical conditions. A heightening of mood (euphoria) is the most common concomitant of altered consciousness, but flattening of mood has also been reported in encephalitis lethargica while depression is not uncommon in the early

stages of both intracranial tumours and tuberculous meningitis. This subject will be dealt with more fully in the next
section of this chapter.

Aggressiveness. 'Behaviour disturbances', especially in children, very frequently accompany disorders of sleep. The fact
that children who recovered from the Spanish 'flu epidemic of
1917 (encephalitis lethargica) very frequently grew up to show
uncontrolled outbursts of aggression is well known. Clardy
and Hill (1949) studied the sleep patterns of children with no
history of cerebral injury but whose behaviour problems had
led to institutionalization, and found a markedly abnormal
number of sleep disturbances amongst them characterized by
restlessness and nightmares.

Physiological mechanisms in altered consciousness

In the clinical material discussed in this section, note has
already been made of the point that cerebral lesions causing
impairment of consciousness tend to be subcortical, within
the limbic system and centred around the mid-brain, the
diencephalon and the reticular formation (mesodiencephalic
activating system) (see Figure 2). Further evidence that sleep
is controlled and mediated by these areas comes from the
experimental work on animals conducted by Magoun and his
associates (see Oswald, 1966, pp. 25-30) and from a study of
human beings born with only the mid-brain and thalamus,
who Cairns (1952) describes as follows:

Some of these individuals may survive for years, in one case of
mine for twenty years. In them, the cerebral cortex is absent or has
virtually disappeared, and the brain-stem and sometimes the
thalamus remain relatively intact. From these cases, it appears that
the human brain-stem and thalamic 'preparation' sleeps and wakes;
it reacts to hunger, loud sounds and crude visual stimuli by movements of eyes, eyelids and facial muscles; it may see and hear; it
may be able to taste and smell, to reject the unpalatable and accept
such food as it likes; it can itself utter crude sounds, can cry and
smile, showing displeasure when hungry and pleasure, in a babyish

way, when being sung to; it may be able to perform spontaneously crude movements of its limbs (Cairns, 1952).

While lowered consciousness is associated with lesions in and around the mid-brain causing impaired activity of these areas, there is also evidence that over-arousal is due to altered activity within the reticular system (Hutt *et al.*, 1964)

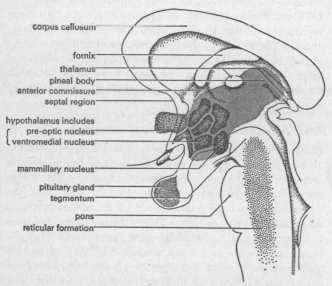

Figure 2 The diencephalon (shaded area) and posterior part of the fore-brain

and there is some evidence that, in animals, behaviour disturbances of the type associated with disordered consciousness may arise from experimental lesions in the ventromedial area (see Herberg, 1967, p. 105). Herberg suggests that these latter findings indicate that the hypothalamic excitatory drive mechanisms are normally opposed by inhibitory mechanisms sited in the ventromedial area of the brain.

The manner in which these areas interact with the cortex and thereby influence mental activity has yet to be established.

From EEG records it seems fairly clear that full alertness is accompanied, not just by response to external stimuli, but also by 'responses to responses' (see chapter 5), and it is possible that from studying these we may learn more about it.

Disorders of Mood

Fluctuations of mood in relation to changes in both physiological and psychological conditions are completely normal and probably vital. It is when mood does not reflect these changes but remains fixed at either too high a pitch (mania) or too low (depression) or fails to move at all (flattened) that it is said to be abnormal. For instance, if the thought of winning the football pools does not make a person feel elated or the thought of the loss of a near relative does not make him depressed, a person's mood is said to be abnormal.

Disorders of mood will be considered here under three sections: (a) the psychological changes accompanying them; (b) the physiological changes accompanying them; and (c) response to treatment.

The psychological accompaniments of mood disorder

A depressed person does not just feel sad, full stop! His sadness usually colours his reactions to all other events and particularly to the way in which he regards himself and his own deeds. He may feel that he is unworthy of the things he has and of the people around him. He may feel that the whole world is heading for destruction, and that he himself is responsible for all that has gone wrong in it. He may even feel that his body is contaminated. In the same way the manic person often projects his sense of well-being and happiness into all he does. He dresses in flamboyant clothes. He goes out and buys unnecessary objects – usually in duplicate or triplicate. He throws his money around feeling that he will never need it again, that a power greater than himself will look after him. He feels filled with unaccustomed strength, is convinced that he can carry out great deeds, that he has been chosen for rare honours, and that his intellectual powers are better than they ever were. It is a common finding, however, that a patient's intelligence and memorizing ability is in direct contrast to his subjective judgement when mood is disordered. The depressed patient, although he feels himself to be incapable and may take time to think out a problem or to recall a past event, is still able to function at a higher intellectual level than the manic patient who thinks himself to be so wonderful but usually functions at a very low level of efficiency.

Physiological accompaniments of mood disorder

Motor. One of the most striking and consistent accompaniments of a depressive state is psychomotor retardation – a slowing up of reaction time, a reluctance to act and a paucity of the actions made. Conversely in the manic state reaction time is shortened and there is an abundance of (often irrelevant) motor behaviour. These alterations are particularly common in the sphere of spontaneous speech, and may even precede the onset of subjective and objective mood changes. Thus one patient who showed marked and regular mood swings was studied over a two-month period by Hutt and Coxon (1965). She showed quite consistent changes in both the speed of her spontaneous utterances and the length of sentence uttered, and the changes in these measures not only correlated closely with her mood but also preceded by a few days each mood swing.

Autonomic activity. Inability to sleep, loss of appetite and a decrease in sex drive are frequent accompaniments of both heightened and lowered mood, although less often seen in the reactive than in the endogenous depressive states. It is a further characteristic of endogenous depression that the mood follows the diurnal rhythm, the patient frequently reporting that he feels worse in the morning and better towards evening.

Factors affecting mood disorder

Since the essence of a mood disorder is its failure to respond to environmental changes, or to psychological pressures, it is not surprising that attempts to alter it by manipulation of the environment or by psychological methods are usually ineffective. On the other hand, disorders of mood do often respond dramatically and gratifyingly to electrical stimulation of the brain and to pharmacology.

Convulsive therapy was first introduced by von Meduna in 1933, following observations that schizophrenic patients often became accessible and tractable after induced seizures. The clinical agents used by von Meduna in the early days were replaced in 1937 by electric currents passed through two electrodes placed on the forehead, an innovation due to Cerletti and Beni. While relieving the schizophrenic symptoms to some extent, however, the effect of this treatment on depressive states is far more dramatic and electric convulsive treatment (ECT) is now used almost exclusively for this purpose.

The usual method of administering the treatment is described in most psychiatric textbooks. Briefly, alternating electric current of 70 to 120 volts is applied through temporal electrodes for 0·3 to 0·6 seconds, the aim being to produce a clinical seizure with the minimum amount of electric current. Treatments are usually given two to three times a week for two to four weeks depending on symptoms. While this treatment is very effective in relieving endogenous and precipitated depression, one serious disadvantage is that it leaves the patient temporarily confused and amnesic. The comparison between the effects of shocks administered bilaterally with those administered unilaterally has been investigated in a number of recent projects. Lancaster, Steinert and Frost (1958) compared the effect of unilateral ECT applied to the non-dominant hemisphere in twenty-eight patients, with the conventional bilateral treatment in fifteen patients, and found that whereas the unilateral treatment certainly cut down the incidence of confusion and amnesia, improvement of the depression was slightly greater and more complete in those who had received bilateral treatment. Later workers, however, did not substantiate this finding and believed that there was no significant difference in the therapeutic effectiveness of the two forms of treatment. Summarizing several papers published between 1960 and 1967, Halliday *et al.* (1968) state:

An important outcome of these results is that they establish that the therapeutic effect of ECT on depression is not directly linked with the degree of memory impairment as has sometimes been suggested. In this connexion, Ottoson's careful study has indicated that in conventional bilateral ECT the memory impairment is probably related to the amount of current flowing through the brain tissue, while the therapeutic effect on depression depends on the occurrence of an epileptic fit.

It has already been pointed out that disorders of consciousness are closely related to lesions in and around the brain-stem. Are alterations of mood due to disturbances in the same area? This question is difficult to answer. Where disorders of mood accompany epilepsy the lesions, where known, usually involve the amygdaloid nucleus and the temporal lobe. This observation has led to suggestions that the amygdaloid nucleus acts as a switch generating emotional activity to the motor system. Since the cerebral areas particularly affected by ECT are not easy to identify with precision, our main evidence on this point comes from the studies of animals in whom electrodes have been implanted by surgical means, and which receive a short burst of electrical stimulations each time they press a bar. The animals soon learn that bar pressing leads to such stimulations, and will avoid or press the bar depending, it is presumed, on the pleasure or pain they receive from doing so. With electrodes placed in the posterior part of the hypothalamus (except for the mammillary bodies) (see Figure 2) bar pressing rates are high. An animal allowed to stimulate itself will continue to do so at the rate of 4500 times an hour, showing no satiation with the passage of time. As the electrodes are moved forward into the anterior hypothalamus and tegmental hypothalamus the rate of self-stimulation begins to decline. 'Rates rise again slightly in the pre-optic region and posterior fore-brain, but they are not as high as in the posterior hypothalamus, and they fall sharply to about 200 an hour as the electrodes are moved forward into cortical parts of the rhinencephalon' (Olds, 1958).

While these findings point to a 'pleasure centre' in the posterior hypothalamus in rats, the extent to which self-stimulation is carried out depends largely on the animal's internal environment. The changes of self-stimulation rate under conditions of hunger and endocrinological disorders are very complex and depend on both the strength of current and precise electrode placement. Concluding his account of a long series of experiments, Olds states: 'When a series of animals was tested for both hunger and androgen effects, we found a remarkable negative correlation. When androgens improve response rates, hunger often had a detrimental affect. When hunger increased response rates, the performance of the same animal was often impaired by the high androgen levels' (Olds, 1958). Injections of chlorpromazine and LSD also have different effects according to the electrode placement; chlorpromazine abolishes self-stimulation only if the electrodes are placed in the posterior hypothalamus and the anterior septal region, while the effects of LSD are most pronounced in some parts of the septal region, but are abolished by preliminary injection of serotonin 'except if the electrodes are deep in the fore-brain just beyond the anterior commisure'.

Chemotherapy. Although this book cannot consider the part played on mental activity by biochemical factors, enough has been said in the last few paragraphs to indicate the likelihood of pharmacological agents affecting the functions of the hypothalamus and so affecting mood. This is indeed the case. While ECT is a very effective (and possibly the only effective) agent in relieving depression in a number of patients, radical relief of symptoms can also be achieved in many by appropriate drugs.

The chemical formulae of the effective compounds are described in a number of textbooks, and the part they play in the cycle of events occurring in the transmission of nervous impulses is also fairly well established; but how these alter a person's mood and how this in turn affects his beliefs, thoughts and preoccupations, we are still far from understanding.

Conclusions

In this chapter it has been pointed out that consciousness and mood are not only influenced by physical events occurring in the brain, but that the areas of the brain most closely involved are closely related to one another and are situated along the brain-stem and in the diencephalon but may also involve the amygdaloid nucleus. Whether mental behaviour is directly due to activity within these cerebral areas or is due rather to the activation of the cortex by them is less clear.

It has also been pointed out, however, that the relation between mood, consciousness and brain-stem activity is complex. It is not simply a question of the more stimulation the better. Overstimulation causes as much discomfort and disruption of mental processes as understimulation; blocking of sensory input is often as vital to effective survival as reaction. Indeed as one famous anatomist said many years ago: 'The main object of the synapse is not to assist transmission but to block it.' While most clinicians regard the main function of the cortex as reacting *to* external stimuli, it may be that this is not the whole truth. It may be that what the alert wakeful cortex is also doing is playing the part of a complicated synapse – delaying the response until after a number of different sensory impressions have been processed. The intimate connexion between consciousness, wakefulness, mood and memory, however, suggests that before speculating any further on the physiological basis for the first three of these states, it would be wiser to consider the fourth, memory.

2 Disorders of Memory

Defects of memory (amnesia) are a common symptom of cerebral disease. As a transient phenomenon they occur in a wide variety of diseases, both those intrinsically cerebral and those of a more generalized nature affecting the brain directly. They are often but one part of a more widespread cerebral dysfunction such as is manifested in diffuse intellectual impairment, delirium, stupor or coma. Sometimes they are the predominant, and occasionally the only recognizable features of the dysfunction (Whitty and Lishman, 1966, p. 72).

Whitty, in the above paragraph, outlines the range of problems confronting the psychologist in this sphere. In order to classify the data psychologists have usually tried to concentrate on answering two questions:

1. What aspects of the memory function are affected by what organic conditions?
2. What areas of the brain are involved?

Classical psychology divides memory into three stages – registration, retention and recall or recognition – but where memory defects are present it is often difficult if not impossible to say in which of these stages the breakdown has occurred. Efforts to overcome this difficulty by re-naming the stages consolidation, storage and retrieval (perhaps to fit in better with computer analogies) have not fully overcome the difficulty, and indeed it will be argued towards the end of this chapter that such a distinction is not very useful and may even be misleading. Clinicians usually prefer to consider memory defects from the point of view of: *anterograde amnesia* – the difficulty of learning new skills and of retaining events that occurred after the onset of the amnesic period; and *retrograde amnesia* – the difficulty of recalling events preceding the onset of the amnesic period.

In this chapter the behaviour of patients in both these conditions will be described and attention will then be paid to the anatomical lesions associated with them.

Anterograde Amnesia

Although the first clinical descriptions of acute or isolated disorders of memory are usually attributed to Korsakov in 1889, Talland (1965) and Zangwill (1966) in their excellent historical reviews both note that even earlier writers had remarked on the existence of such clinical states. The condition described by Korsakov and which now bears his name includes among its symptoms, disorientation and confabulation as well as inability to retain information, but it is only the latter which will be considered in this section. The condition presented by such patients is described and analysed in detail by Talland (1965) in a group of chronic alcoholics, by Milner (1966) in a patient with bilateral mesial temporal lobe resection, by Williams and Pennybacker (1954) in a series of patients with tumours involving the third ventrical and by Williams and Smith (1954) in patients with tuberculous meningitis. Anterograde amnesia is also well known as a transitory state following concussional head injuries, as well as after ECT administered therapeutically for the relief of depression.

Milner describes one patient who had undergone temporal lobe resection for the relief of epilepsy as follows:

He could no longer recognize the hospital staff, apart from Dr Scoville himself, whom he had known for many years; he did not remember and could not re-learn the way to the bathroom, and he seemed to retain nothing of the day-to-day happenings in the hospital. . . . Numerous illustrations of the severity of the amnesia could be given. Although he mows the lawn regularly, and quite expertly, his mother still has to tell him where to find the lawn-mower, even when he had been using it only the day before. The same forgetfulness applies to people he has met since the operation, even to those neighbours who have been visiting the house regularly for the past six years. He has not learned their names and he does not recognize any of them if he meets them in the street (Milner, 1966, p. 113).

Talland subjected a group of sixteen patients who showed chronic Korsakov states to a carefully controlled series of tests concerning reasoning ability, perception, learning and recall. On tests of intellectual and perceptual ability, and on tests of immediate recall, these patients did not show any marked deficit. It was only when the tests involved the serialization of data that defects were evident. In summarizing their performance, Talland (1965) states:

The patients are able to form new associations, but, once established, these dissolve very rapidly. Practice by repeated exposure or repetition does not advance their learning, and neither does the correction of errors. Multiple associations with the same response creates special difficulties; spatial cues can be helpful. While some verbal associations may last for an hour or even longer, conditioned responses extinguish almost instantly. . . . If Korsakov patients learn but little when instructed to, their incidental learning is scarcer still. Neither old nor recent learning seems to transfer in their formal tests of learning, although they can apply old skills to novel situations and tasks, especially if these involve simple routine operations (p. 232).

The learning defect noted in such patients, nevertheless varies to some extent with the nature of the task. Talland's patients were able to acquire manipulative skills to a limited extent even though they were quite unable to learn the solution to spatial puzzles or to acquire verbal passages. In the latter, forgetting seemed to involve: 'Sheer loss of information, not just a distortion of the content. They learn or retain emotionally loaded reports no better than neutral accounts' (p. 256).

Amnesic states similar to the ones described above may be seen following concussional head injuries, in some infective disorders (tuberculous meningitis), in association with certain intracranial tumours, and following ECT, for the treatment of depression. This last condition allows for more experimental study and will be considered in some detail.

The usual method of administering ECT has been described on p. 29. Ever since ECT was first used, it has been noted that an adverse effect on memory is an almost invariable sequel. For some time after the fit and before full orientation is established, patients pass through a confusional period very similar to that following concussion. At this time they tend to be disoriented and to forget sensory impressions as soon as the stimulation is withdrawn. The extent, duration and severity of the post-ECT amnesic symptoms are found to vary with different individuals and to depend on a number of factors such as the time after treatment at which memory is assessed, how it is assessed (i.e. by recognition or recall) and the nature of the stimuli the subject is asked to remember. However, in the post-ECT amnesic state, as in other organic amnesic states, the after-effect of experience may often be seen in some form even though this may be difficult to categorize as 'memory'.

In two series of experiments conducted on subjects in the post-ECT confusional period, Williams (1950) showed subjects a number of visual stimuli (pictures) and recorded their responses to them. It was found that:

1. The appropriate name for a picture could be elicited at its second appearance with less intensive stimulation than at its first appearance.

2. On the first occasion the appropriate name was often preceded by inappropriate verbal responses ('approximations') and these were also elicited by less stimulation the second time than the first, i.e. the whole sequence of behaviour leading up to correct naming was repeated but was triggered off more easily a second time than a first.

3. Priming of a behavioural response (naming) by eliciting it in one context, e.g. by one picture, resulted in it being given more often and more quickly on later occasions and in response to other stimuli. This is in contrast to the behaviour

of normal people, who, if they give a certain verbal response to one stimulus are *less* likely to give it to a second dissimilar one ('That's not as good a tree as the other was').

These points seem to suggest that in the amnesic state, behavioural responses can be facilitated by prior arousal, but that they are not associated with the type of sensory image which constitutes the full aspects of a memory. Moreover, the emotions aroused by a stimulus may persist and become associated with other stimuli whilst the original stimulus is forgotten (Williams, 1952).

The effect of applying the electrodes to one side of the brain only (unilateral ECT), has been described in a number of papers (see also p. 29). In a systematic study carried out by Halliday *et al.* (1968), fifty-two depressed patients for whom ECT had been prescribed were randomly assigned to one of three treatment groups. The first received a standard course of four ECTs at half-weekly intervals administered bilaterally with conventional bifrontal electrodes. The second and third received the treatment unilaterally to the right or left hemisphere only. All the patients were under sixty-five, right-handed, without sinistrality in the family, and had no evidence of organic brain disease. Before ECT was started, the patients were given four memory tests involving: (a) immediate memory (digit span); (b) a verbal learning (word association) task; (c) a non-verbal learning task (Rey Davis) in which the position of four fixed pegs had to be identified in an array of thirty-six similar but movable ones (Williams, 1968); and (d) a test of delayed recall (pictures).

The patients were re-tested half a week after the fourth ECT had been given, and again three months after the termination of treatment. Half a week after the fourth ECT, verbal learning was selectively impaired in those who had received ECT to the dominant hemisphere, and non-verbal learning was impaired in those who had received ECT to the non-dominant hemisphere. Bilateral ECT produced an intermediate pattern of impairment. After three months the verbal memory impairment was still present in the patients who had received dominant hemisphere ECT, but the impairment of non-verbal memory appeared to be more persistent following bilateral ECT than following unilateral ECT to the non-dominant hemisphere.

Further discussion of the part played by the two hemispheres in the memory process will be delayed until later.

Categorization of the defects seen in anterograde amnesia shows them to fall into two main groups – learning and remembering.

Learning

Although as already described, amnesic patients have particular difficulty in acquiring new skills, certain aspects of learning are retained.

Retention of acquired behaviour patterns. It has long been recognized that although some hospitalized patients with chronic amnesic states might deny that they had been in their wards for more than a few hours, they nevertheless behave therein as if they knew exactly what to expect and where to go. If asked to show the way to their beds they would do so without error (maintaining if questioned that these were only the beds they would sleep in if they were to stay). Talland found some evidence of the ability to acquire manipulative skills in his Korsakov patients and Williams (1960) also found that senile patients with severe memory disorders could be 'trained' to run simple finger mazes without error although they usually denied after short time intervals that they had ever seen the tasks before. Milner's patient described on p. 34 showed progressive improvement in a mirror-drawing task over successive days (judging by reduced time and error scores) although he never remembered each day that he had done the task before. Similarly, considerable improvement both within trials and over successive days in the ability to recognize incomplete words and pictures was found in six amnesic patients by Warrington and Weiskrantz (1968).

Improvement over successive trials on a learning task can often be seen in the attempts of these patients to acquire behaviour patterns (as mentioned above) although in many cases there may be little residue the next day. For example, a patient in the amnesic period following tuberculous meningitis was able to learn the Babcock sentence ('One thing a nation must have to become rich and great is a large, secure supply of wood') after three attempts, but had no recollection of having heard it the next day (Williams and Smith, 1954).

Immediate reproduction of a given stimulus (e.g. digit span) shows little impairment in these patients.

Remembering

The difficulties inherent in judging whether an event has been remembered or not are well known to psychologists. The main changes which occur with the passage of time in all memories are:

1. Displacement in time and place. We remember having visited a place or having met someone, but exactly when it was and just where we were at the time is often harder to establish with certainty.

2. Partial recollection. One may remember part, though not the whole of an event or scene. Some aspects of it stand out while others are blurred.

3. Distortion. In remembering an event or stimulus we are inclined to distort the original. We remember a thing as we would have liked it to be, rather than as it was. An ambiguous figure may be given a name and then made to look more like the object named. An asymmetrical one becomes more symmetrical during repeated reproductions.

4. Condensation. Parts of the original experience may be left out and other parts altered, until the whole is condensed into a small, meaningful unit.

5. Closure. Pieces may be added to an incomplete figure to make it fit more easily into a frame of reference.

The recollections of amnesic patients show all the above

changes and depend on the same conditions as the recollections of normal subjects. Descriptions of these conditions can be found in most psychological textbooks, and can be summarized briefly as follows:

1. Time lapse. The greatest loss is seen in the first few minutes after an experience, but occasionally there is a re-awakening of memories which are not recovered immediately – reminiscence.

2. The nature of the stimulus. Pleasant events, those carrying some degree of affect, familiar ones, or uncompleted ones, are less quickly forgotten than their opposites.

3. The manner of presentation. A set to recall is of paramount importance. Events which a subject knows he will be expected to remember are better preserved than others.

4. Events during the retention interval. The more fully the interval has been filled, the less a person is likely to remember of events preceding it. The more closely subsequent events approximate the one a person is trying to remember, the worse is likely to be his remembrance.

5. The manner of testing – in particular the amount of reinforcement ('prompts') provided.

6. The individuality of the subject – in particular his age, intellectual ability and cultural upbringing.

Conditions 2–6 affect the remembering of amnesic patients in much the same way as that of normal subjects; it is the effect of time lapse (1) which distinguishes the amnesic from the normal person. Reminiscence rarely occurs in amnesic patients (although apparently forgotten items can often be re-awakened by prompts).

Retrograde Amnesia

Retrograde amnesia in chronic amnesic states

In conjunction with anterograde amnesia, patients with organic memory disturbances very often have difficulty in recalling events which preceded the onset of the amnesic period – retrograde amnesia. These events, which were well recorded at the time, tend to be forgotten in inverse relation to their recency and led Ribot to postulate his famous 'law of regression' (Ribot, 1885).

For example, Milner's patient referred to above, 'did not remember the death of his favourite uncle three years before, nor anything of the period spent in hospital before the operation, but did recall a few trivial incidents that had taken place just before his admission to hospital. His early memories were seemingly vivid and intact' (Milner, 1966, p. 113). A patient described by Talland 'was oblivious of everything since the time he had run a farm, long before his admission to the hospital at the age of 78.'

In these patients, the loss not only covers recall of events and incidents, but may include generic images. Thus Zangwill (1950) describes a patient who, when asked to draw a public transport vehicle and a lady in modern clothes, produced illustrations of both dating from some fifteen years before the onset of his illness.

Retrograde amnesia after concussional head injuries

Retrograde amnesia not only follows chronic and irreversible conditions such as those mentioned above, but a gap for past events may remain in patients who have suffered from head injuries long after recovery of all other mental functions. Broadly speaking, it has been found that the extent of the amnesia varies considerably at different stages of the illness and may be very much greater at the height of the illness than after recovery. This 'shrinkage' of amnesia in the course of recovery has been described by many authors (Russell, 1959; Symonds, 1937, Williams and Zangwill, 1952). It is often believed (see Russell, 1959) to occur in order of relative time sequence, i.e. the more remote events in memory being restored first, again following Ribot's principle, but exceptions to this are extremely common. Williams and Zangwill (1952) carried out a careful study of thirty-two cases of head injury. The patients were observed from an early stage after admission until the time of discharge from hospital. Follow-up studies after discharge were carried out wherever possible. Three grades of severity of head injury were arbitrarily defined on the basis of duration of the post-traumatic-confusional state, and hence of the duration of the post-traumatic amnesia as assessed after full recovery. In group 1 (nine patients), duration of post-traumatic amnesia was under one hour; in group 2 (nine patients) it was one to twenty-four hours; and in group 3 (fourteen patients) over twenty-four hours.

In group 1 the patient's 'last memory' after recovery of normal consciousness referred to an event which had preceded the moment of injury by under ten seconds (five cases) or by ten to thirty minutes (four cases). In the former cases there was always some haziness or amnesia for earlier events which cleared up rapidly over the next few hours or days. The order of recovery of memories, however, was not always in inverse ratio to their recency. In the latter cases there was progressive recovery of memory for events which had occurred both before and after that represented by the patient's 'last memory'. Again, no very clear direction of shrinkage could be ascertained.

In group 2, the pattern of recovery of pre-traumatic memory as a rule followed that displayed by the four cases in group 1 who had presented islands of recent memory. In group 3, the study of recovery of memory was found to be complicated by defects in associated mental fields, especially by confusion, impaired conceptual grasp, memory defect for current events, disorientation and confabulation. It is seen from these cases, however, that recovery from amnesia is shown not merely in the ability to recall more and more recent events with increasing ease or clarity; it involves above all the recall of events in orderly sequence, and the rebuilding of a coherent background of past experience. Although there is some tendency for the most recent events to be most often forgotten and to be restored latest, there are many exceptions to this principle. Availability of an event in memory is not wholly a function of its recency, and memory defects can be shown in ways other than in availability to voluntary recall. Russell (1959) has drawn attention to the fact that 'visions' for isolated events falling within the retrograde amnesia can occasionally be found during the early post-traumatic stages when the patient is still confused and amnesic, but not be recalled after full recovery. This suggests that some forgetting due to time lapse may occur during the time the patient is in post-traumatic amnesia and that, as well as shrinkage, retrograde amnesia may show some extension due to lack of rehearsal, a point which will be taken up again in the discussion at the end of this section.

Some studies of the residual *retrograde memory defects* seen after recovery from head injury, when retrograde amnesia has attained its final brief and static duration, have also been reported (Russell, 1959; Williams and Zangwill, 1952).

Williams and Zangwill's main findings were:

1. Some degree of residual memory defect (outside the short retrograde amnesia) for quite recent events preceding the head injury was found in a majority of cases submitted to careful psychological interrogation. This defect took the form of an actual memory gap, of hazy and ill-defined recollection or of errors in temporal reference. The phenomena observed are very reminiscent of those found in the recall of relatively remote events in normal individuals.

2. The more severe the head injury, the more likely were residual memory defects to occur.

3. The defects were apparently irreversible in the group of twenty-four cases studied.

In the light of these findings, it may be surmised that the process of shrinkage analysed in the earlier paragraphs is often less complete than is frequently supposed. Further, it may be suggested that the length of memory gap preceding the impact (retrograde amnesia in the conventional sense) is not necessarily a guide to the completeness of restoration of recent memory.

An important point to note is that retrograde amnesia is rarely, if ever, seen without some degree of post-traumatic amnesia (see Table 1). This is to say that unless the stream of consciousness is interrupted for at least some minutes, no preceding memory gap remains.

Table 1

Duration of Post-Traumatic and Retrograde Amnesia Compared in 1029 cases of 'Accidental' Head Injury (Gunshot Wounds Excluded) (Russell, 1959)

Duration of RA	Duration of PTA						
	Nil	1 hr	1–24 hrs	1–7 days	7 days	No record	Total
Nil	99	23	9	2	0	0	133
Under 30 min.	—	178	274	174	80	1	707
Over 30 min.	—	3	16	41	73	0	133
No record	—	4	14	14	15	9	56
Total	99	208	313	231	168	10	1029

Retrograde amnesia after tuberculous meningitis

Much the same picture may be seen in patients after tuberculous meningitis as in those after head injuries. As in the head-injury cases it is found in many patients after tuberculous meningitis that apparently permanent retrograde memory defects are in evidence after otherwise complete recovery. These memory defects may extend over very long time intervals preceding the onset of the illness. As in the case of head injuries they are also far from complete losses of memory. For example, a soldier who was interviewed two and a half years after making a good recovery, had little recollection of the two years preceding his illness except for one or two isolated events. He remembered that he had been posted to a regiment in the Ruhr where he took a clerks course. He learned typewriting and apparently became very efficient; but he found that on recovery from his illness all that he could recall of the course was a large plaque on the wall, the first letters of which were QWERT. Later he was shown a photograph of the men on the course. He found that he could name them all without difficulty, although he would have had no idea when or how he had met them (Williams and Smith, 1954).

Retrograde amnesia after ECT

The retrograde amnesia caused by ECT allows for a more methodical examination of the defects than is possible in most clinical material, and this opportunity has been exploited by psychologists, in both animals and men. Although most patients usually deny any recollection of visual stimuli presented to them within a few seconds before the onset of the seizure, it has been noted that such stimuli can frequently be 'picked out' on a choice recognition test (Mayer Gross, 1943) or can be recalled with prompting (Williams, 1950). Material learned by repetition is affected in the same way as isolated stimuli, but the nature of the material and the ease with which it is originally learned, affects the degree to which it is subject to retrospective inhibition from ECT. As in normal people, that which is learned easiest is remembered best.

Although retrograde amnesia in animals cannot be studied in the same detail as in humans, i.e. the difference between subjective and objective memory disturbances cannot be ascertained, work with animals allows for greater control of the variables than it does with man. The effect of electric convulsive shock (ECS) on behaviour established prior to it has been studied in a number of experiments (see Weiskrantz, 1966). The procedure is usually to follow a single unique experience, such as stepping down off a raised platform, with an unpleasant experience such as electric shock to the feet. Rats learn avoidance (not to step down), with ordinary subconvulsive shock in one trial. With convulsive shock as the only consequence of stepping down, they learn to avoid only very slowly with repeated trials, but they do definitely learn, particularly when the interval between the response and

ECS is very brief. The apparent amnesia for the electric shock is affected by: (a) the time elapsing between ECS and the retest; and (b) the number of times the animals are replaced in the original setting (equivalent perhaps to the number of cues provided for recall in the human situation) (Zinkin and Miller, 1967).

Comparison between amnesic defects and normal forgetting

Since the events which are or are not recalled in organic amnesia depend so much on personal interest and on contextual reinforcement, it is not surprising that organic disorders are difficult to distinguish from those of psychogenic origin, or that the two often fuse together. Cases in which an organically induced amnesia has been attributed to 'malingering' and vice versa are, indeed, not hard to find in the literature. One of the most famous and best documented controversies raged over a case first described by Grünthal and Störring in 1930 and recently analysed again by Zangwill (see Zangwill, 1967).

It has sometimes been suggested that the rapid loss of information occurring in anterograde amnesia is due to the poverty with which perceptional stimuli are absorbed or integrated in the first place.

In almost all the human subjects who demonstrate anterograde amnesia, it is true that some degree of mental disorder outside the sphere of memory can usually be demonstrated. Thus the patients are typically somewhat euphoric, lacking in initiative and disinclined to attend to their environment with the same intensity as normals. Nevertheless, many of them carry out the usual intelligence tests with above the average ability and compared with control groups of patients show no evidence of impaired perception or reasoning. Experimental work with animals rules out perception itself as being a cause of the memory defect. Wilson and Mishkin (see Weiskrantz, 1966) showed that monkeys with lesions in the visual cortex managed to learn visual pattern discrimination better than those with inferotemporal lesions, despite having considerably greater loss of vision. Moreover the defects seen in both animal and human studies only appear with the lapse of time. Tests carried out within a very brief period of learning (such as those of immediate reproduction – e.g. digit span) usually show no decrement, once again indicating good preservation of perception and (temporary) assimilation.

These observations might lead, and have led, observers to conclude that the defect in anterograde amnesia lies merely in retention, or the transference of short-term memory traces to long-term memory traces. But if this is accepted, where does short-term memory end and long-term memory begin? Moreover, when a stimulus cannot be recalled spontaneously, but can be recovered in response to prompts, is it to be regarded as in the short- or long-term memory store? Finally, why can some things be retained and others not? How is it that easy associations are better retained after ECT than more difficult ones, or that motor skills are better learned by Korsakov patients than verbal ones?

These points will be returned to later. For the moment it is sufficient to point out that whatever the problems posed by memory in general, anterograde amnesia shows much the same process as normal forgetting but occurs much faster. A rather different problem is posed by retrograde amnesia, especially by the short retrograde amnesia which follows a head injury or ECT. Retrograde amnesia seems to defy the laws of normal forgetting in that remoter events tend to be better remembered than recent ones while the residual memory gaps are not recovered in response to cues or any other form of prompting. Some form of consolidation of a memory trace would seem to need to be invoked to account for it and has, indeed, been invoked on many occasions.

In order to investigate further the difference between normal and abnormal memory for isolated events such as those forgotten in retrograde amnesia, the present author undertook two investigations. In the first, twelve patients who had not been subjected to head injury or any other cerebral insult, were asked to describe a number of events in their past lives. In the other investigation patients who were having ECT were shown pictures within seconds of the application of the current but were warned beforehand that they would be asked about the pictures later, i.e. given a 'set' to remember.

In the first investigation the subjects consisted of twelve patients – six who had been admitted to hospital for illnesses of sudden onset (perforated ulcers, fractures, etc) and six who had been admitted for illnesses of more gradual onset. Half of the patients in each group were interviewed the day after admission to be comparable with head injury patients suffering short retrograde and post-traumatic amnesias; the other half were interviewed two to three weeks after admission to be comparable with the more severe head injury patients.

Each subject was asked to describe (a) how he had spent the previous twenty-four hours; (b) how he had spent the last two hours before admission to hospital; (c) how he had spent some important day in his remote past, e.g. his wedding day.

It was noted that there was a big difference between the subjects' accounts of recent and remote events and of those preceding sudden trauma, and those preceding illness of gradual onset. Those preceding sudden trauma were recounted as sequences of isolated acts in which equal weighting was given to all events. For example, one patient in this group, describing the morning before an accident, said: 'At 8.30 the alarm went and I made a cup of tea. The post arrived at 8.54. Then I let the dog out. . . .' The events of his remote past were organized into meaningful and coherent schemes in which individual happenings could be 'supposed' or 'guessed at' in recall. 'I know I *must* have had breakfast on the day I got married,' said one patient, 'but I can't really remember eating it.'

It is concluded that unless a comparatively routine and unimportant event is followed by some catastrophe which causes its rehearsal, it normally becomes schematized and confused with other past memories. Thus events which are not followed by something which encourages rehearsal tend to drop out in the normal course of time. This conclusion is supported by the report of one patient who had broken his leg falling off a motor cycle, and was able to describe in detail the antecedent events: 'I always mend my own punctures, and had just mended one that day. I suppose I must have bungled it as going round a sharp corner the tyre burst – and that was it.' Asked when he had mended the puncture previous to this and what had happened subsequently, he looked quite offended and remarked, 'How could I possibly remember that, nothing happened to fix it'.

In the second investigation the recollection or recognition of pictures by seventeen ECT patients who had been warned that recall would be expected of them (primed group) was compared with that of seventeen patients who had not been so warned (unprimed group). Recall of each picture by the thirty-four patients was scored according to the following scheme: (a) the picture could be drawn accurately and named; (b) the picture could be picked out on a recognition test; (c) the patient remembered having been shown a picture but did not recognize it; and (d) the patient had no recollection of having been shown a picture.

The number of responses scored in each of these categories by the patients in each of the two groups is shown in Table 2. Although the differences just fail to reach a significant level

Table 2

Showing the Grade at which Pictures Immediately Prior to ECT were Recalled by Primed and Unprimed Patients

Grade of memory	Number of subjects	
	primed group	unprimed group
a	7	4
b	8	7
c	1	1
d	1	5

(Mann–Whitney U-Test) the number of responses falling into categories (a) and (d) in the two groups are strikingly different.

It has frequently been remarked that retrograde amnesia only occurs after some degree of post-traumatic amnesia (Russell, 1959), and it has further been established that the longer the post-traumatic amnesia, the longer tends to be the retrograde amnesia (see Table 1, p. 44). This, and the evidence put forward in the two investigations just quoted, suggest that forgetfulness for the events preceding a head injury may be accounted for primarily by non-rehearsal. It is the *desire* to recall them which is the abnormality. Those events which are forgotten, would have been forgotten in the normal course of events without a head injury, unless they had been rehearsed as a result of some ensuing catastrophe. It is not necessarily the interruption of the traces but the interruption of rehearsal which is the cause of the gap in memory.

Amnesia in childhood

This subject has never been described in detail in any publication, but most clinicians are familiar with its occurrence. The defects are essentially similar to those seen in the adult but must be assessed against a background of normal memorizing ability. The immediate memory span and ability to acquire new skills increases with age in childhood, so that mental age can be assessed by the amount and complexity of material a child can reproduce immediately after a single hearing. Retention of visual and non-visual skills also shows increase with age but as against this the ability to localize and recognize discrete visual stimuli (Kim's game) possibly reaches its optimum at the ages of eleven to fourteen, and begins to deteriorate at the same time that the reproduction of discrete experiences tend to be confused by 'sets' and expectancies derived from past experience.

It is particularly, therefore, in its effect on the recollection of discrete visual stimuli that amnesia in childhood can best be recognized. The responses of children to the test situation are, however, somewhat different to that seen in adults. Children with fewer past experiences and established habits or skills to fall back on are less inclined to confabulate when pressed for recall than are adults. They tend, instead, to remain mute. If given a prompt or a cue, children respond in a less related way to it than adults, and if forced to make a response may repeat what they have just done or heard instead of falling back on past personal idiosyncrasies (Table 3).

Table 3

The Different Responses Shown by Amnesic Adults and Children in a Memory Test Situation

Adults	Children
Reluctant to admit inability	Readily admit 'I forget'
Respond to cues by some act related to cue	Respond to cues by some act often unrelated to cue
Repeat past individual habits or skills	Repeat last act done or last thing heard

The extent to which acquired skills (such as learned tasks) may be lost by children in amnesic states has not been clearly established. It is possible, for example, that the muteness of the amnesic child may be partly caused by his having forgotten how to speak.

The difference between the child and the adult is restricted to the response pattern. The factors affecting recall are the same in children as in adults and need not be listed again here.

Psychological mechanisms

In trying to define memory the main problem is to explain how a short-term memory trace becomes a long-term one. While 'schematization' is a useful word to describe the process, the actual stages involved in the process are still somewhat obscure. Some psychologists prefer to use terms such as 'coding' or 'transferring encounters into rules', but these are still only expressions of the problem rather than solutions to it. Can the study of amnesia provide any help in this direction?

It has been argued here that the breakdown of memory seen in clinical conditions seems to be mainly an accentuation of the normal process of forgetting which occurs with time lapse. Even the retrograde losses due to head injury and ECT, it has been argued, are similar to those which occur with the passage of time alone; but the clinical conditions do indicate two points which do not appear to have been fully considered by experimental psychologists.

1. Since learning in one sensory modality or of one skill may break down independently, it follows that not all aspects of memorizing can depend on a single function. For example, organic patients frequently do very well on tests of immediate memory retention but poorly on those of delayed recall. They can repeat a past response although the stimulus originally arousing it leaves no sensory impression. The mood aroused by an event may persist after the event itself is forgotten.

2. Memory is not an all-or-none affair; memories occur in different grades of accuracy which might themselves be subject to measurement and should be taken into account when the process itself is being considered. Thus the memory of an event which is recalled in its full and original context with all its original clarity, is a very different experience from one which is recalled 'as in a dream'. These differences and a number of intermediate stages can be clearly recognized in the clinical setting.

The physiological mechanisms responsible for the various mental processes covered by the term 'memory' must now be considered.

Neuropathology

A thorough but selective review of the evidence associating amnesic defects with cerebral lesions has been made by Brierley (1966), as a result of which he concludes that

the structures essential for the process of normal memorizing are the hippocampal formations within the temporal lobes, the mammillary bodies and possibly certain thalamic nuclei within the diencephalon.

The anatomical connexions of these two regions suggest that a continuous pathway might be traced along the afferent fibres from the hippocampal gyrus to the hippocampus and out, via its efferent pathway the fornix, to the mammillary bodies. From these, the mammillothalamic tract leads to the anterior nuclear complex of the thalamus, which projects to the cingulate gyrus. The pathway is completed by the known connexions between the cingulate and hippocampal gyri. This apparently continuous 'circuit' lies within the group of structures comprising the 'limbic lobe' to which Papez ascribed the elaboration of emotion and the control of visceral activity (p. 173). (See Figures 3 and 4.)

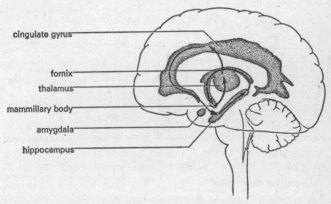

Figure 3 The main structures in the limbic system containing the circuit of Papez

In coming to these conclusions (which are shared by the majority of other authors), Brierley considers only those cases which presented clear-cut, isolated and well-documented memory disturbances, and well-defined and isolated cerebral lesions. Thus cases with widespread vascular or neurological involvement have not been included. Brierley divides his material into two main groups:

1. Lesions in the mammillary bodies and the thalamus usually showing a full Korsakov psychosis and predominantly due to metabolic disorders or dietary (vitamin B) deficiency but may also be due to intracranial tumours.

2. Bilateral lesions of the hippocampal formation usually resulting from surgical intervention for the relief of epilepsy or psychosis. One of these latter cases, Scoville and Milner's patient, has already been referred to in this chapter. In these cases bilateral re-section of the uncus and amygdaloid nucleus (see Figure 4) alone do not appear to cause amnesia, while unilateral interference causes only defects in the verbal skills if carried out in the dominant hemisphere, and passing and subjective sensations of forgetfulness if confined to the non-dominant hemisphere.

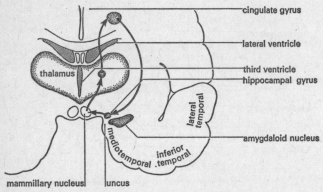

Figure 4 Mammillothalamic tract in transverse section

Brierley's memory circuit has long been generally accepted as connected with memory functions, yet as he himself points out:

The most discrete anatomical link between the hippocampal and diencephalic regions is the fornix. It is surprising, therefore, that with the exception of the case reported by Sweet, Talland and Ervin, bilateral division of the fornix (usually in the region of the intraventricular foramen)[1] has not resulted in a disorder of memorizing. This finding suggests that the two groups of structures linked by the fornix cannot be regarded as a unitary system subserving the

1. See Figure 1 (p. 18) for the positioning of the intraventricular foramen.

process of memorizing, at least until major interconnexions other than the fornix have been identified (1966, p. 173).

Experimental work on animals has only added to the uncertainty rather than clarifying the issue. Monkeys on which temporal resection was carried out were retested by Cordeau and Mahert (1964) three to four years post-operatively, and were found to have shown a remarkable degree of recovery. Those which had undergone removal of the inferior temporal area were still poor on visual retention tasks, but this was attributed to defects of discrimination rather than retention, for they showed no impairment on auditory retention tasks. Those with laterotemperal ablation showed the opposite discrepancy, but those with mediotemporal lesions showed full recovery in both modalities. These authors suggest that damage to the amygdala–hippocampus complex may have only a temporary effect.

The circuits postulated above are only put forward to account for the retrieval phase of memory. Where and how the events themselves are stored is another problem. Some form of trace storage at least within the cerebral hemispheres seems to be demanded by the evidence of the 'split brain' studies which have been carried out in the past few years. Steele-Russell and Ochs (1963) developed a technique for putting one hemisphere out of action while leaving the other functionally intact. If the animal (a rat) was trained on a task, and then retested with the trained hemisphere inactivated but the previously inactive one functioning, it was unable to carry out the task, and could only do so when the trained hemisphere was again functioning. The behaviour of humans in whom the two hemispheres have been surgically divided to prevent the spread of epileptic activity also show features suggestive of some form of memory storage. Skills carried out by one hemisphere cannot, in these circumstances, be elicited by stimuli applied to the other (Gazzaniga and Sperry, 1967). More will be said of this later on. These findings, however, do not tell us at all where or how the memory itself is stored. Lashley (1950) finally gave up the search for the 'engram' and, like others in this field, concentrated on explaining retrieval only. But not everyone has held this line. Explanations in terms of synapse alteration and cell conductivity have been put forward, and since 1947 a new possibility has been discussed – that the cell protein structure acts as a template for the synthesis of protein replicas.

How these units might function is a problem neuropsychologists enjoy discussing at length. Many models have been put forward, one of the most intriguing, perhaps, being that based on the analogy of the hologram. Pribram (1969) describes this as follows:

In a hologram, the information in a scene is recorded on a photographic plate in the form of a complex interference or diffraction pattern that appears meaningless. When the pattern is illuminated by coherent light, however, the original image is reconstructed. What makes the hologram unique as a storage device is that every element in the original image is distributed over the entire plate. ... If even a small corner of a hologram is illuminated by the appropriate input, the entire original scene reappears. Moreover holograms can be layered one on top of the other and yet be separately reconstructed.

Pribram suggests that, similarly, in the brain, images may be produced by wave fronts travelling along neural networks that set up interference patterns with other wave fronts. He suggests that the function of the cortex is merely that of organizing the processes of assimilation and reconstruction. However, as yet, this, like other models, is merely an analogy.

Conclusions

At the end of the last chapter, the part played by the brain in mediating consciousness, wakefulness and mood was considered. It was suggested that activation of the cortex by the brain-stem actually retards rather than facilitates the immediate response to individual stimuli, and thereby allows for a response to be influenced by previous habits based on past experience – memory.

In this chapter it has been pointed out that, like consciousness, memory can be considered on a number of different planes and as affecting a number of different functions. For a sensory impression to leave the sort of trace which can affect consciousness as defined before, it must be integrated with other sensory impressions and these integrations must be rehearsed (i.e. repeated in the mind) a number of times. Nevertheless, the traces so formed are unstable. They are subject to alteration by all later stimuli, and it is this alteration which is known as forgetting.

After lesions around the brain-stem and diencephalon, forgetting is particularly quick. These are the same lesions which affect consciousness. In the case of memory, however, the mammillary bodies, the hippocampus and the fornix also seem to be involved; and since many cases have been recorded of patients who, although being alert, fully orientated and capable of advanced intellectual activity, forget an incident or event as soon as it has passed, it may be the function of these latter areas which are mainly responsible for retention. Smythies (1966) suggests that, whereas the amygdala–hypothalamus system is the area which determines what memories shall be laid down, it is the hippocampus–fornix system which is responsible for their preservation.

Since memory involves the integration of sensory stimuli, the next area to consider is this latter function itself.

3 Disorders of Perception

Although it is never easy to distinguish between a disorder of simple sensation and one of perception (i.e. the interpretation of a sensation), this chapter will attempt to deal mostly with the latter. It is certainly true that many of the perceptual disorders which follow cerebral injury are accompanied by, and may to a large extent be dependent on, sensory deficiency; yet the fact that they are also seen in the apparent presence of full sensory function and in a setting of clear consciousness has been recognized for many years.

Agnosia, as these perceptual disorders are called, occur primarily for *visual*, *auditory* and touch or *proprioceptive* stimuli – the latter causing *disorders of the body image*.

Visual Agnosia

Visual agnosia is frequently seen in conjunction with loss of sensory input such as blind-spots (scotomata) and defects of the visual fields due to injury of the optic tracts. However, the perceptual defects so often noted in organic conditions can seldom be attributed entirely to the sensory deficits. The defects consist not so much in non-awareness of the stimuli as in misrecognition of their meaning. Objects, faces, spatial configurations, pictures and colours lose their sense of familiarity. Although each of these defects can occur in isolation (and will be dealt with in this chapter as if they did so), it is more usual for a patient who shows difficulty in recognizing one type of stimulus to have difficulty in recognizing others, too.

Visual object agnosia

'A sixty-year-old man, almost blind in his right eye from an old injury, woke from a sleep unable to find his clothes, though they lay ready for him close by. As soon as his wife put the garments into his hands, he recognized them, dressed himself correctly and went out. In the streets he found he could not recognize people – not even his own daughter. He could see things, but not tell what they were' (see Critchley, 1953, p. 289). This case first described by Bay in 1952 is an excellent example of a patient with visual object agnosia, a condition which had been recognized in dogs by Munk in 1877 and described in humans by Stauffenberg in 1914 and Goldstein and Gelb in 1918 (see Critchley, 1953, p. 276).

It is usually noted that patients with visual object agnosia can recognize objects by touch although the ability to recognize them by their visual contours appears to be very largely lost. Although defects of visual acuity are not always present it has been argued that, in the majority of cases showing visual object agnosia, perceptual disorders are also present in other spheres. Indeed, Gloning, Gloning and Hoff (1968) found only three cases of visual object agnosia among the 241 patients studied by them, and in each of these cases the symptom was accompanied by a variety of other perceptual disorders.

Prosopagnosia

Prosopagnosia or the inability to recognize faces, while frequently seen in all patients with visual agnosia, has been held by some authors to occur in isolation. Bodamen describes one patient to whom faces appeared

strangely flat; white with very dark eyes, as if in one plane, like white oval plates ... all the same. He could see but not interpret facial movements and grimaces. . . . Gazing in a mirror, he described the delineaments of what he saw, but could not recognize the face as his. Together with three other soldiers, he had his photograph taken, but he afterwards failed to recognize his face in the print. The features of his closest relatives, either in snaps or in real life, appeared quite foreign to him. He walked past his mother in the street, and he never got to know the looks of the other patients in the ward (Critchley, 1953, p. 293).

The connexion between prosopagnosia and other forms of visual agnosia has been debated at length. While some observers believe that recognition of facial configurations is a specific act, and that it can be disturbed when all other visual functions remain intact, others regard it as only one aspect of the visual recognition process. Thus Warrington and James (1967b) found some difficulty in the recognition of faces (from photographs) in sixty-two patients with unilateral cerebral lesions (those with lesions on the right side being worse than those with them on the left), but they were inclined to regard prosopagnosia as merely one constituent of an amnesic syndrome. De Renzi, Faglioni and Spinnler (1968) agree that prosopagnosia 'represents simply the most prominent aspect of a generalized visuo-perceptual disturbance' (and also that it occurs more frequently in right- than in left-sided brain damage), but also follow other observers (Gloning, Harb and Quatember, 1966; Gloning et al., 1966) in pointing out that for the recognition of faces it is necessary to fixate and synthesize certain key parts – especially the eyes. If such fixation is difficult for a patient (one quoted by Gloning, Gloning and Hoff, 1968, described how the eyes of people he looked at seemed to be 'strange and permanently changing'), facial recognition is likely to be impaired.

Colour agnosia

An artist quoted by Holmes, 'no longer was able to use colours after he had sustained a stroke. He was not colour blind, however, for he could name most colours and pick out colours correctly to command. He could not associate colours with objects except by reference to rote memory' (see Critchley, 1953, p. 276).

Another patient studied in detail by Stengel (1948) had difficulty in both matching and naming colours.

When requested to pick out coloured skeins to match the colours of an object named by the examiner, he succeeded as a rule, but not without considerable hesitation. In this test, too, differentiation between green and blue were the most difficult. Which colour is a pillarbox? 'It would be a blue with a red – post-office red'. (Patient picks out a brown-red skein first then a bright red.) Grass? (Patient picks out light green.) Sky? (Patient picks dark green.) Blood? (Correct.) Tomato? (He hesitates, points to purple, then to orange, adding that the latter was more likely to be correct.)

In assessing colour agnosia it is important to make full allowance for the possible presence of dysphasia (see chapter 4), for patients who have lost the ability to recognize or say words can often give a most misleading impression. Indeed colour agnosia and word-blindness often occur together (Gloning, Gloning and Hoff, 1968), and it seems quite possible that the patient described by Stengel above was suffering more from misrecognition of words than of colours.

This does not mean that the patients cannot often express themselves quite lucidly. Critchley (1965) analyses the features of colour agnosia which distinguish it from true colour blindness of peripheral origin. In colour agnosia the colour boundaries of objects seem to be distinct from the form boundaries, sometimes shimmering, fluctuating and even spreading to other areas. Critchley, in a review of the subject which stretches far beyond the immediate clinical environment, discusses this point in relation to the use of blue in the history of art and the development of language! He points out that in painting, blue only appears fairly recently as an object-identifying colour, and that a specific word for this colour appears later than for most others in the language of different cultures.

Alexia, the difficulty in recognizing words and letters will be dealt with in the section on speech (see chapter 4).

Simultanagnosia

This consists of inability to absorb more than one aspect of a visual stimulus at a time (Weigl, 1964, Wolpert, 1924). For example, a sixty-eight-year-old right-handed patient studied by the present author had difficulty finding his way around because 'he couldn't see properly'.

It was found that if two objects (e.g. pencils) were held in front of him at the same time, he could only see one of them, whether they were held side by side, one above the other, or one behind the other.

Further testing showed that single stimuli representing objects or faces (including pictures) could be identified correctly and even recognized when shown again, whether simple or complex (newspaper photographs or simple sketches). If stimuli included more than one object, one only would be identified at a time, though the other would sometimes 'come into focus' as the first one went out. If the stimuli were placed side by side, the right one was usually identified first, gradually giving place to the one on the left. Single letters were identified correctly, especially when in the right visual field. Those in the left visual field were sometimes neglected, sometimes over-elaborated (P became B) and just occasionally fused with the one on the right. If long sentences were presented, only the most right-sided word could be read. If sentences were short, the right-hand words would be read first followed by those to the left of it. Thus 'the dog runs' was read as 'run dog'. If single words were presented, these were read without error. If a single word covered as large a visual area as a sentence which could not be read, the single word was read in its entirety, but a double-barrelled word was misread, only the last syllable being identified, even though the first part might leave some impression. Thus to the word 'houseboat' the patient said, 'I see boat – but *not* houseboat.'

If the patient was shown a page of drawings, the contents of which overlapped (i.e. objects drawn on top of one another), he tended to pick out a single object and deny that he could see any others. Moreover the figure selected at the first exposure of such stimuli was the only one seen on all subsequent presentations. If shown a drawing which might be seen in two different ways, and which to the normal person usually appears first in one configuration and then in the other (reversible figures), he would pick out one configuration only and was quite unable to reverse it.

This condition, first described by Wolpert in 1924, has led to considerable discussion, Kinsbourne and Warrington (1963a) studied three cases of simultanagnosia on the recognition of visual stimuli shown tachistoscopically. They found that whereas the recognition time of the first of any two successive stimuli was always within normal limits, there was invariably long delay to the second. If pairs of stimuli were shown together, the left was always seen before the right (in contrast to the case mentioned above). They believe this delay to be the basis of the disability – a conclusion also reached by Birch, Belmont and Karp (1967) who found that if two stimuli were presented at time intervals differing by 300–600 milliseconds both could often be identified together.

Although the condition of simultanagnosia bears some resemblance to the difficulties experienced by a normal person in a situation of stereoscopic rivalry (i.e. when trying to fixate a different stimulus with each eye), it is different in that there is less fluctuation between perceptions in simultanagnosia than in the stereoscopic situation. Nevertheless, some of the conditions affecting dominance of perception in stereoscopic conditions might well be studied for their effect in cases of simultanagnosia. Is one item more likely to be seen than another if it is brighter, simpler, the right way up, meaningful, or emotionally loaded? (See Rommetveit, Toch and Svendsen, 1969.) These points have not been studied.

Simultanagnosia is somewat similar to *visual inattention* though the latter is seldom recognized unless specifically looked for. In this condition the patient tends to recognize only one object if two are held up in different visual fields; that is to say he ignores the second object unless his attention is specifically drawn to it. Unlike patients with simultanagnosia, however, the patient who shows visual inattention is usually capable of seeing the two objects once his attention is drawn to them.

There is a tendency for patients to neglect the left side of visual space more than the right, just as they tend to neglect the left sides of their bodies more than they do the right and, if asked to draw or copy pictures, they will very often omit the left side or cram all the details of it onto the right of their paper. This tendency is usually attributed to the fact that visuo-perceptual disorders appear to be associated with lesions in the right parietal area and so affect the functions of the left half of the patient's body.

Metamorphopsia

Although this is a defect of experience rather than of perception, metamorphopsia is usually considered alongside the agnosias.

In this condition objects may be recognized accurately but are subjectively distorted – either larger (macropsia) or smaller (micropsia), tilted (when walking one patient felt as though the pavements sloped to her left), inverted, fragmented, drifting, a long way away, or unfamiliar. Examples quoted by Critchley are as follows: 'the furniture seemed to be turned round'; 'my husband seemed too big and yet a long way away'; 'people's faces would frequently change, their eyes would swell and contract ... they looked terrible. The eyes go to nothing at all then come back like a pimple.'

Despite the nature of these distortions the patients can usually recognize and name the things which seem so strange to them. There is not so much agnosia for the objects as distortion of their visual contours.

Apart from the inability to recognize individual items as described above, other disturbances in the visual sphere include the following three.

Visual perseveration

Occasionally visual perceptions may seem to continue for an abnormal length of time (paliopsia), as after hashish and mescalin intoxication; or to recur after the stimulus object has been removed. Thus, 'after a person had walked past the foot of the bed from left to right and then had gone away, she had a moment or two later the impression as if the same person had walked past as before' (Critchley, 1953, p. 304). The special conditions associated with visual perseveration in one patient were studied in considerable detail by Kinsbourne and Warrington (1963b).

Denial of blindness

Denial of blindness (Anton's syndrome) could be regarded as a special form of visual perseveration in which a visual image appears so clearly to the patient who has no visual perception at all, that he may maintain volubly that he can see all that is around him. If asked to describe a picture held by the examiner (who is holding nothing) he will confabulate freely. This condition is not common. Out of 708 patients with verified cerebral lesions, Gloning, Gloning and Hoff (1968) found only eleven cases, and in ten of these there was also gross confusion. These authors, in fact, tend to attribute the symptom to loss of criticism, euphoria and a tendency to fabricate in general.

Occasionally the denial applies to a blind half-field only, the patient describing all the things he imagines to be present in it. Warrington (1962) has shown that a tendency to do this occurs in the majority of patients with left-sided, visual field defects, but King (1967) has pointed out that such completions tend to be common only on symmetrical figures where 'expectation' could give rise to the same sort of phenomenon as is common in the normal overlooking of a printer's error.

Visuo-spatial disorientation

Visuo-spatial disorientation refers not so much to the misrecognition of objects as to their mislocalization in space. Patients have difficulty telling which of two things is above or below the other, which is nearest or further away, which is to the right or the left. A case described by McFie, Piercy and Zangwill (1950) 'began to leave food on the left side of her plate or to push it off on to the table. In reading she experienced difficulty shifting down to the next line. About the same time, she began to have great difficulty in finding her way about in places she knew well. This improved slightly but the patient noticed great difficulty in learning her way around in a strange house.'

The defects in these cases are most obvious if the patients are asked to draw either from memory or from models shown to them. As will be described in greater detail in chapter 4, they have particular difficulty in combining parts of objects into coherent wholes, in joining diagonal lines and in filling out the left side of a page.

Psychological mechanisms

Whether all the above phenomena can be attributed to a single basic disorder or whether each has its own specific mechanism cannot be decided on the basis of the information available to date, but a number of possible 'basic mechanisms' have been postulated and will be considered here.

Faulty visual sensation. It has already been mentioned that visual agnosia is not dependent on loss of visual sensation. The two may be connected in some instances – e.g. Warrington (1962) found that completion of missing parts was more often carried out in the absent visual field than in the intact one – but neither partial nor total blindness in themselves produce any of the symptoms mentioned in this chapter. Critchley has made a careful comparison between the performance of blind and agnosic patients and noted that the blind experience none of the spatial disorientations so commonly seen in patients with agnosia.

Faulty visual scanning is a commonly evoked basis used to explain visual object agnosia. Bay, himself, tends to accept this explanation. He observed how one patient would enter a room cautiously, peering around and turning his head from one side to the other. He did not fixate objects normally and would readily deviate his eyes towards any new stimulus. Abercrombie (1960) has certainly found evidence of grossly unsteady eye movements in cerebral palsied children, correlating with their poor performance on visuo-constructional tasks.

It is also interesting to note that while omissions or neglect are almost always made to the left side of visual space, experimental work has shown that normal subjects tend to show a less pronounced but similar tendency, recognizing pictures and objects in the right half of visual space better than those in the left. This observation suggests that the defect in brain lesions may be an accentuation of a normal tendency.

The tendency for normal adults to scan systematically from left to right (thereby fixating more strongly on the right) has often been attributed to reading habits. Ghent–Braine (1968) studied Israelis with a view to seeing whether subjects whose reading habits had taught them to scan from right to left showed this same tendency. However, her work does not completely solve the problem. Whereas the adult subjects studied by her did recognize patterns shown to them tachistoscopically better on the left than on the right, as predicted on the hypothesis of a learned scanning pattern, the difference only became evident in those who had attained at least the seventh grade of reading. Previously to this the right field predominated over the left, suggesting a more fundamental physiological basis for right visual field preference than mere habit formation – a suggestion substantiated by Orbach (1967) who also studied Hebrews and found that right-handed Hebrew subjects showed an even more marked tendency in this direction than left handers.

Insufficient integration of the scanned parts has also been suggested by Gloning and others (Gloning, Harb and Quatember, 1967; Gloning et al., 1966) to account for some instances of prosopagnosia. Scanning defects, however, could not alone account for simultanagnosia or for visuo-spatial disorientation, in which conditions it is not the realization of the parts which appear to be lacking but the ability to see them as a whole. Moreover, faulty visual scanning has been identified by Luria, Karpor and Yarhuss (1966) in patients with frontal (as opposed to parietal) lobe lesions, but in such patients leads to 'impulsive hypotheses about the contents of visual stimuli' rather than to the types of disorder that have been outlined here.

Faulty visual imagery is another postulated causal factor in visual agnosia. Loss of visual imagery plus loss of dreaming has been described in three cases of brain damage due to gunshot wounds by Humphrey and Zangwill (1952). But in the majority of patients who show visuo-spatial agnosia there appears to be no difficulty in visualizing the objects which the patients are trying to reproduce. They know what they want to draw, they can see them in their mind's eye. It is the execution which is at fault.

Slowed-up processing of visual data has been suggested by Kinsbourne and Warrington (1963a) as a basis for simultanagnosia and by Birch and Belmont for visual extinction. Whether such a process could be demonstrated in the other forms of visual agnosia mentioned here, such as object agnosia, prosopagnosia etc., is uncertain and never appears to have been investigated. The mechanism postulated by Kinsbourne and Warrington seems to have a parallel in the changes which occur in normal ageing. Thus Wallace (1956) found that while older subjects were nearly as good as younger ones at identifying simple visual displays, there is a progressive age decrement as the material becomes more complex. This is attributed by the author to the increased time taken to integrate stimuli by older subjects.

Faulty integration does indeed seem to be the only factor common to all aspects of visual agnosia – but having said this has one said anything at all? Until we know what the processes are which underlie or constitute integration of sensory stimuli we have only given another name to an observed phenomenon. It is true that the more items a subject has to integrate into a single percept (e.g. the complexity of the task) the more clearly his disabilities are shown up. The integration of input from two different modalities is often more difficult than the integration of many items from a single modality. Thus Ettlinger and Wyke (1961) report a careful study of one patient with visual object agnosia whose touch-recognition was actually retarded when he was allowed to add visual to his tactile information.

Careful analysis of the conditions which do and do not assist behaviour in the brain-injured patient, together with a study of the stages through which normal performance is attained, appears to be the best hope of gaining insight into the problem. Reference has already been made to some work in this area in the section on visual scanning as an explanation of neglect of the left side. It was suggested by this work that neglect of the left field so frequently seen after brain damage is merely an accentuation of a normal process resulting from the scanning habits developed through reading. Another parallel between normal and abnormal behaviour was shown by Ettlinger (1960) who compared the performance of brain-injured with normal subjects on a picture recognition task. Thus pictures shown tachistoscopically were recognized by the normal subjects before they could be fully interpreted, indicating that recognition precedes – and is therefore independent of – interpretation in normal subjects. It is not, therefore, surprising that it should break down after the latter in cases of brain damage.

In conclusion, it seems that two processes may be at fault: (a) the speed with which sensory data are assimilated, and decoded; and (b) the amount of sensory data which can be processed (i.e. integrated with other data) at any moment in time.

Physiological mechanisms

Visual agnosia is closely associated with lesions in the parieto-occipital area (see Figure 5). About this there is little controversy. But the extent to which lesions in the different hemispheres cause different types of disorder is still debated.

The hemispheres have traditionally been considered as dominant (or major) and non-dominant (or minor). The major hemisphere is that which controls the preferred hand and, since the neural tracts connecting the brain and the limbs cross over in the brain-stem, this is the hemisphere contralateral to the hand used for such specialized tasks as writing. In right-handed people, the left cerebral hemisphere is dominant, and vice versa.

A suggestion that lesions in the minor hemisphere might cause greater disorders of visual perception than those in the major one was, when first put forward, greeted with some

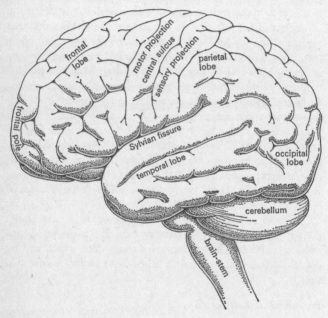

Figure 5 The cerebral lobes

scepticism. At that time all the higher mental functions were, like language, supposed to be carried out by the major hemisphere, the action of the minor hemisphere either being negligible or merely supportive.

The role of the non-dominant hemisphere in perceptual processes has, however, been studied extensively in recent years by neuropsychologists. McFie, Piercy and Zangwill

(1950) published a series of eight cases in which gross visuo-spatial disorders were observed and in whom 'the lesion was exclusively or predominantly right-sided'. Critchley (1953) analysed the localization of nineteen cases in which visuo-spatial disorders were not complicated by disorders of language. Eleven were solely in the right hemisphere, seven were bilateral and only one (unverified) was in the left.

Gloning, Gloning and Hoff (1968) have published a large and well-documented series of cases showing that disorders of visual perception are predominantly associated with lesions in the right parietal area in both right- and left-handed patients. Critchley draws attention to the possibility that in left-sided lesions, disorders of language may somewhat obscure the picture and that, in left-sided cases, spatial disorders may not be absent so much as secondary to those of speech. In this connexion Humphrey and Zangwill (1952) report an interesting case of a left-handed man with a right occipito-parietal gun-shot wound. This patient showed all the usual symptoms of visuo-spatial agnosia (with severe neglect of the left side) and a minimal loss of verbal fluency.

Further evidence that the right hemisphere may control spatial functions, in the same way that the left controls verbal ones, comes from the number of reports comparing the WAIS sub-test performance of patients with unilateral lesions. The common finding is that in patients with left-sided lesions the verbal scores are inferior to the performance ones (the latter depending primarily on the manipulation of visual data), whereas in right-sided lesions the opposite is the case (McFie, Piercy and Zangwill, 1950). Warrington and James (1967a) tried to define the actual functions carried out by the two hemispheres more clearly by studying groups of patients with localized lesions on a task of picture recognition and on the Gollin (incomplete) figures. They found that on the picture recognition task those with left-sided lesions made errors of naming while those with right-sided ones made errors of recognition. On the Gollin figures, those with right-sided lesions were worse than those with left. Where patients with left-sided lesions did make mistakes, these were usually associated with poor performance in other perceptual tasks. These authors argue from this that perception and recognition are two distinct activities. Kimura (1963), however, suggests that true recognition of visual data may involve some aspects of verbalization. Studying patients with right and left temporal lesions on the perception of visual stimuli presented tachisto-scopically, she found that the patients with right-sided lesions were inferior only to those with left on the recognition of unfamiliar material, and suggested that the disability of vision seen in right-sided lesions only becomes apparent when verbal identification is lacking. In support of this suggestion, Kimura (1967) found that when normal subjects are shown visual stimuli in one visual field only (see Figure 6), letters are recognized better in the right than in the left and non-alphabetical stimuli better in the left than in the right. This finding, however, seems to depend to some extent on cerebral dominance, for McKinney (1967) found that in left-handed normal subjects the same lateralizing difference is not so apparent as in right-handed ones.

Warrington (1969) has discussed the whole subject in detail in her consideration of constructional apraxia, but agrees with the general conclusion that although much confusion still seems to exist regarding the functions involved in visual perception in general and in the activity of the two hemi-spheres in this skill in particular, the right hemisphere does seem to contribute more than the left to the perceptual com-ponents of skills. Semmes (1968) has put forward a neat model to account for the difference between the right and left hemi-sphere functions. She suggests that in the left hemisphere focal representation may favour integration of *similar* units, thus giving rise to fine sensory motor skills and speech, whereas in the right hemisphere integration may consist of *dissimilar* units, accounting for multi-model co-ordination. Whether these two different systems can actually be verified at a neuro-anatomical level remains to be seen.

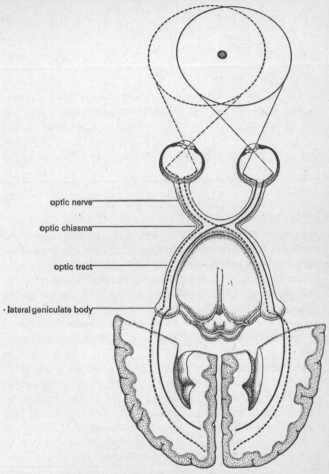

Figure 6 The visual pathways and projections of the visual fields onto the occipital cortex

Disorders of the Body Image

Although disorders of the body image are not outstandingly common – even in parietal lobe lesions – they are common enough to have been recognized for many years and to be described in most text books on neurology. A body-image disturbance consists either of the patient's unawareness of part of his body or of a misconception of its position. There is general agreement that such disorders are associated with (a) an abrupt lesion, (b) clear consciousness and (c) some motor weakness. Except where special techniques of investigation are described the disturbances are usually elicited by observation or simple interview.

The main disorders can be listed and described as follows.

Unilateral neglect

A patient with no serious weakness will sometimes ignore one side of his body (usually the left) or fail to carry out commands with it. When asked to lift his arms, he lifts one arm only. When dressing, he puts on only one shoe or combs only one side of his hair. This condition can be demonstrated by the 'glove test'. The examiner tosses a pair of gloves into the patient's lap, telling him to put them on. The patient commonly puts on only one (usually the right hand) leaving the other aside.

Two points to note in this condition are that:

1. The neglected half of the body functions quite well in spontaneous, automatic acts, and those in which the two sides of the body have to be co-ordinated (e.g. in the glove test, the neglected hand is used to place the glove on the accepted one).

2. While the accepted hand often crosses the midline of the body to help on the neglected side, the opposite seldom occurs.

Patients showing neglect often also demonstrate a curious indifference about it. They appear unconcerned if the condition is pointed out to them, and although not euphoric will cheerfully laugh at themselves.

Anosognosia

Anosognosia might be regarded as an extreme form of neglect in which the patient not only fails to recognize his disability but actively denies its existence. Thus if asked to lift his paralysed arm, the patient either moves the intact one and maintains that he has carried out the command, or if prevented from doing this will lie immobile and after a few seconds mutter, 'Well, there you are, that's done.'

In some cases the paralysed limb may be repudiated or attributed to the presence of someone else. One patient quoted by Critchley always referred to her hemiplegic leg as 'Toby'; another seen by the present author maintained that her own body was perfectly intact and that the hemiplegic limbs at her left side belonged to her husband.

Illusions of corporal transformations

These are sometimes seen, patients reporting that the shape of their bodies are changing or that the size of certain limbs have shrunk or become enlarged. Such sensations are usually transitory and frequently follow focal seizures.

Finger agnosia

Finger agnosia consists of doubt and hesitation concerning the fingers only. This is a special and often isolated form of body-image disturbance whose association with right–left disorientation, agraphia and sometimes acalculia and colour agnosia was first noted by Gerstmann in 1924. Existence of the symptom may be elicited in a number of ways.

1. The patient may be asked to name a finger touched by the examiner (*E*).

2. The patient may be asked to hold up a finger named by *E*.

3. The patient may be asked to point to a named finger on *E*.

4. The patient may be asked to carry out complex commands such as 'put the third finger of the right hand on the tip of the second finger of the left hand'.

5. The patient may be asked to point to the finger on a chart which *E* touches on him.

6. The patient may be asked to touch or name on *E* the same finger which *E* touches on him.

It is usually found that the same errors are made on both hands, but that subjects do better on some of the tests than on others, i.e. they have greater difficulty in indicating fingers than in naming them (apraxia) or vice versa (finger aphasia). It is also commonly noted that more errors are made on the two middle fingers (third and fourth) than on the thumb, index or little finger.

Finger agnosia may occur in the absence of any other form of body-image disturbance, and it is worth noting that agnosia for the toes is very rare indeed.

Phantom limbs

Supernumerary phantoms. While phantom limbs are almost invariably experienced by all subjects at some period after an amputation, they are less rarely but still occasionally experienced by subjects in association with hemiplegic limbs. In the latter cases, the phantom limb is usually supernumerary to the healthy one and usually refers to the fingers of the hand, less commonly to the upper arm and very rarely to the lower limbs. The phantom limb appears to mirror movements carried out by the normal one and tends to vanish as soon as the hemiplegic limb is moved or located visually. Total hemiplegia of the affected limb is not essential. Walshe describes a patient who 'would imagine that his left arm was behind his back as if the two hands were clasped; that is, as if he were a soldier standing at ease. His immediate impulse was always to grope and determine the whereabouts of his real arm in case he should accidentally hurt it. As soon as he found the arm, the phantom feeling would disappear' (see Critchley, 1953, p. 243).

The vividness of supernumerary phantoms can, according to Critchley, 'be manipulated pharmacologically. It can be restored after spontaneous disappearance by mescalin, and it can be oblated by cocainization of the real limb' (1953, p. 244).

Phantoms resulting from actual amputation can also recur after cerebral lesions. L'Hermitte (see Critchley, 1953) describes an interesting case of one patient whose left leg had been amputated at the thigh some years before and who subsequently developed a left hemiplega following a cerebrovascular accident. After this the patient not only denied the amputation but insisted that he had an intact and useful left leg which he could see and feel. One patient seen by the present author, who lost his right leg in the Second World War and whose phantom had since disappeared, had a renewed appearance of the phantom in association with right-sided Jacksonian epileptic attacks.

Phantom limbs following amputation. The association between the disorders described above, the normal body image and its development allow for much discussion and speculation. A good deal of information regarding the normal body image comes from the study of phantom limbs which, as already mentioned, follow the sudden loss (usually through amputation) of limbs with previously normal sensation.

Phantoms following amputation have been noted since the beginning of medical history, but it was Weir Mitchell (Mitchell, 1871) who first established the almost universal occurrence of this phenomenon in adults. The phantom is often so real that a patient on awaking from the operation refuses to believe that a limb has been amputated (Simmell, 1963), but with the passage of time both the vividness and the form of the phantom undergo modification. From a phantom of the whole limb as it used to be (though not necessarily, according to Simmell, in the position it was in at the moment of loss or injury) parts begin to drop out and those that remain become telescoped or smaller in size. It is important to note that the first parts to go are the upper arm and thigh; then follow the lower limb and calf and after them, the knee and elbow. The fingers and toes are the last parts to remain and often feel as though they are attached to the stump. Even in deformed limbs (amputated for aesthetic or practical reasons), it is the terminal parts (hands and digits) which are most strongly represented in the phantom. An interesting point here is that the phantom of the congenitally deformed limb resembles the deformity rather than a normal limb (Weinstein, Sersen and Vetter, 1964). Thus visual influences may play a large part in deciding both the original shape of the phantom as well as in the alterations it undergoes, but there is a close and striking parallel between the importance of a body-part in the phantom and the area of cortex involved in its normal control, as demonstrated by Penfield and Boldrey (1937) and illustrated in their famous homunculus – a point which will be discussed later.

Factors affecting phantoms. The two most common factors affecting phantoms are age at amputation and nature of the limb lost. Simmell (1962) has studied the phantoms of children after limb amputations and has found that the longer the subject has had and used the amputated limb the more frequent and the more persistent is the phantom experienced. Children under four years old seldom claim to experience phantoms and phantoms are never experienced for congenitally absent limbs. On the other hand, phantoms of the sex organs tend to decrease as sexual potency decreases (Simmell, 1963; Weinstein, Sersen and Vetter, 1968). It seems, in fact, that the phantom reflects the degree to which the limb has been integrated into the body image in the past and is a part of current activity.

For a phantom to occur at all, it has been consistently noted that the limb has to have had previously good sensation and be removed suddenly. Those digits which have been absorbed into the body as a result of leprosy do not appear in phantoms but – and this seems to be an important point – if a half-absorbed digit is amputated the full digit may appear as a phantom (Simmell, 1956 and 1961). Explaining this, Simmell (1963) suggests: 'The new schema that has developed as a result of progressive absorption lacks the stability of the earlier schema' and may be superseded by it.

Mechanisms involved in body-image disorders. In trying to account for phantom phenomana and for body-image disorders in general, three different types of mechanisms have been considered.

1. *The dynamic concept* attributes phantom phenomena and anosognosia to the patient's reluctance to admit to bodily loss. Argued forcibly by Schilder (1950), stress is laid on the not infrequent traits of personality disorder which accompany phenomena. Finger agnosia is similarly explained. It is argued that since the hand is the extension of thought into space, the disorder must be primarily mental rather than physical.

While the fact that reluctance to accept disability may be present in most patients showing these defects, there is no evidence that it is not also present in those who do not; and the fact that both anosognosia and finger agnosia are most commonly associated with lesions to the right hemisphere only, is a serious argument against dynamic factors as being solely responsible.

2. *The derivatory hypothesis* attributes body-image disorders primarily to defects in other spheres of mental activity, notably verbalization. Thus Weinstein, Cole and Mitchell (1964) conclude that 'the predominance of anosognosia for the left side is an artefact of the method of study usually employed.' From a close examination of twenty-eight patients with right-sided sensory motor defects, they found anosognosia in fifteen. There was, moreover, an inverse correlation between anosognosia and aphasia, from which the authors argue that anosognosia may occur on the right side just as often as on the left but in these cases is usually hidden by the patient's inability to describe it. They admit that the descriptions by those with left-sided anosognosia 'are in general more bizarre' and are more often associated with unilateral neglect than those on the right, but they attribute the bizarreness to the florid language often used by patients with right cerebral lesions and regard

it as due to a linguistic rather than a perceptual disorder. Thus Weinstein, Cole and Mitchell would tend to avoid a purely organic basis for body-image disorders and, although not as committed as Schilder to a dynamic interpretation, would see it more in terms of a resultant of other disorders.

In this connexion Critchley's analysis of the salient features of Gerstmann's syndrome (agraphia and acalculia with finger agnosia) is interesting and challenging. Asking why the hand should be the most affected body-part, and what its connexion may be with calculating, writing and right–left disorientation, Critchley points out that counting begins – historically as well as in each individual – with the fingers and is still linguistically associated with them. (We call the numbers 1 to 9 the digits.)

The close connexion between verbal, motor and perceptual activity is further emphasized by Halnan and Wright (1961) who, in an amusing but well-presented paper, draw attention to the fact that while the thumb, forefinger and little finger have the largest areas of cortical representation and are also the least affected in finger agnosia, they are also the only digits to have commonly used names in the English language. None the less, perceptual awareness and indeed right–left orientation can occur without their verbal equivalents, and even precede verbalization in childhood. Thus Jambor and Williams (1964) found that for some years before they are able to give directions in verbal terms, children are able to find their way around simple mazes and complex corridors, indicating directions by naming landmarks instead of laterality.

3. *The organic hypothesis* argues that body-image disorders are caused by disruption of the physiological processes carried out by discrete anatomical areas. Strong arguments in favour of this are drawn from the fact that disorders of body image are, with very few exceptions, seen only in association with lesions in the parietal area; that anosognosia is usually confined to lesions in the right or non-dominant hemisphere, and finger agnosia to those in the left or dominant one. From the summaries of twenty-eight published cases of Gerstmann's syndrome reported by Critchley it appears that only five were

in the right hemisphere and amongst these, two of the patients were left handed or ambidextrous (see Table 4). Predominance of left-sided lesions was also found by Gloning, Gloning and Hoff (1968) in their survey of cases with focal cerebral lesions. Of the 241 patients studied by them fifty-three showed some aspects of Gerstmann's syndrome. In forty-nine of these the lesions were in the left hemisphere and, in all except one, were localized in the parietal area. Gerstmann himself was convinced that the lesion responsible for his syndrome lay 'in the region of the parieto-occipital convexity [of the dominant hemisphere], particularly in that part which is represented by the transitional region of the angular and the middle occipital convolutions' (see Critchley, 1953, p. 224).

Table 4
Location of Lesions Associated with Gerstmann's Syndrome
(from data in Critchley, 1953)

| Handedness | Location of Lesions | | |
	L. hemisphere	Bilateral	R. hemisphere
Right handed	18	4	3
Ambidextrous	1	0	1
Left handed	0	0	1

In the case of anosognosia and other body-image disorders, localization of the lesion is less precise. Critchley, in fact, after very careful consideration of the data, believes one can go no further than to relate it to the parietal area in general. To try to localize lesions further he submits would be unjustifiable. To discriminate between superficial and deep lesions or to narrow them down to lesions of a particular gyrus he does not believe to be warranted.

Semmes *et al.* (1963) raise an interesting question of the relationship between disorientation of the body and that for external objects which they distinguish as bodily disorientation and external disorientation. From a study of seventy-six U.S. veterans who had sustained localized gunshot wounds of the brain, they concluded that while there was a close correlation between the two forms of disorientation (independent of other factors such as aphasia or dementia) the two were not related to the same cerebral areas. Left-hemisphere lesions of the anterior parietal area affected personal orientation more severely than external, but right-hemisphere lesions of the posterior area affected external more than personal orientation.

In summarizing the content of this section, one sees that the name usually given to the disorders described here – namely, body-image disorders – is unjustified. The body *image* of these patients is undisturbed. The concept they have of their bodies, the image due to past experience, is still present. It is awareness of the real body and its present position which seems to be at fault. Information relating to the real body is failing to reach consciousness; it is not becoming integrated with other mental acts. The patient is carrying around, as it were, a phantom of himself, and in the absence of severe or prolonged external stimulation, lives with this phantom instead of with reality.

Defects of Auditory Perception

Studies in this field mostly concern the perception of music (amusia) and of language (word deafness). The recognition of other sounds such as running water, a car starting, a telephone bell, etc., have only recently been the subject of very extensive systematic study. In 1966 Spinnler and Vignolo reported an interesting study of patients with unilateral brain lesions who were asked to listen to tape-recorded sounds and match them with pictures of the objects making them. Those patients with lesions in either hemisphere which did not affect speech made no more mistakes than normals; but the patients with speech disorders (dysphasia), especially those showing loss of comprehension, made a significant number of errors.

Another interesting study by Bender and Diamond (1965) concerns the localization of sound stimuli by patients with unilateral lesions. These authors found that the mislocalization of a sound source and a tendency to ignore the stimulus making it, were predominant on the side contralateral to the hemisphere affected. These authors examined patients with known cerebral disorders but no defect in the peripheral auditory system. The defects noted concerned changes in volume, interruption, repetition, reverberation, roughness and garbling of speech or music. All, or some, of these could occur in patients at different times and were very similar to the disorders which can result from peripheral deafness. The most striking disorder in the patients with intracerebral lesions was not in the nature of the disturbances reported but in the fact that these were reported almost always in association with the stimuli arriving in the half-auditory space contralateral to the hemisphere affected. Occasionally stimuli which were presented in the affected half space would be localized in the other half space or would be ignored altogether. These signs were usually transitory and were closely related to other mental impairments (Bender and Diamond, 1965).

The defects of central auditory perception differ from those of peripheral deafness in that:

1. The latter concerns sounds of specific tone or pitch (e.g. high-tone deafness), whereas the former is independent of these factors. Thus, whereas deafness may affect consonants rather than vowels, sensory auditory impairment concerns the meaning of whole words.

2. In central auditory deafness, sounds can usually be heard (and even repeated) but the meaning that these convey appears to be totally lacking.

In both conditions, however, transitional probabilities (see p. 86) and expectancies are usually intact, and in both conditions reading and writing of language may exceed comprehension of the spoken word.

Amusia

Although amusia has been recognized in the clinical field for some time, little systematic study appears to have been made of the conditions involved. For instance, it is not known whether familiar tunes are better recognized than unfamiliar ones, or what the factors involved in musical appreciation and its opposite really are.

It has long been recognized that loss of the ability to understand words is not always accompanied by loss of musical appreciation. This may be due to the fact that the two processes are carried out by different parts of the brain. Indeed, Milner (1962) noted that right temporal lobectomy appears to lead to greater loss of tone discrimination (as measured on Seashore's test) than the same operation carried out on the left side, and a considerable amount of attention has been paid to this field. Further discussion of this topic and its theoretical implications will be left until later in this chapter.

Word deafness

Loss of the ability to understand language can occur in very many different grades, from very severe to very mild. Appreciation and measurement of these depends on special tests, one of the most carefully worked out and clinically useful being that described by Boller and Vignolo (1966). This test was first published in 1962 under the title 'Token Test' (de Renzi and Vignolo, 1962) and consists of nine tokens varying in shape, size and colour. These are placed in front of the subject who is then given a series of commands increasing in complexity from 'touch the red circle' to 'before touching the yellow circle pick up the red rectangle'. This test is put forward as an improvement on the famous Pierre-Marie 'Three-Paper Test', which has been in clinical use for many years. The latter consists of presenting a patient with three pieces of paper and a variety of somewhat complex commands telling him what to do with them. Standards for the Pierre-Marie test have never been established inside or outside clinical practice and scoring procedure is entirely left to the administrator. In the Boller and Vignolo test standards are presented (Boller and Vignolo, 1966) for a number of patients with left and right brain damage including those who do not show any clinical signs of dysphasia. It is found that defects on the test can still be demonstrated with left-hemisphere damage even when clinical signs of dysphasia are completely lacking.

As in all other instances of mental impairment following cerebral injury, losses of verbal comprehension are seldom complete. Under certain conditions some information seems to get through. If the patient can be cued in to the correct concept, he can often recognize the meanings of the words spoken to him. If he is given a limited number of words or pictures to match to sounds, he can often make the correct pairings.

It is typical of these patients that short sequences (i.e. short sentences and single-syllable words) are more easily understood than long ones, and that phoneme distinction follows the same rules as for normal people (i.e. the voiced–unvoiced distinction is the most difficult). It is also frequently found that sudden or irrelevant noises may be completely ignored as if the patient were deaf, and furthermore that the patients may be quite undisturbed by having their own speech relayed back to them after a short delay (delayed auditory feedback) which to most normal people is extremely disturbing.

Word deafness in children. Some children, although not deaf, never apparently learn to understand (or decode) speech. This was first recognized by Worster Drought and Allen in 1928. Since then, word deafness in children has been a subject which has fascinated neurologists but has remained little studied by psychologists.

Care has always to be taken to ensure that children diagnosed as word deaf are not just suffering from inability to hear high-frequency tones, but even when this contingency has been ruled out, there still remain some children who never learn to appreciate spoken language. Ingram (see Gordon and Taylor, 1966) has suggested that this defect may be due to poor specialization of the two hemispheres, and Gordon and Taylor (1966) support this view in suggesting that a maturational deficit underlies the condition. Landey *et al.* (see Gordon and Taylor, 1966) were able to study an autopsy on a ten-year-old boy whose speech comprehension was very slow, and whose brain showed reduction of the gyri in the posterior parieto-temporal and occipital lobes of both hemispheres.

Word deafness and jargon aphasia. The connexion between word deafness and comprehension in jargon aphasia could be discussed at great length and will be referred to again in the next chapter. Here, the point may be made that word deafness may occur in the absence of jargon, and conversely that in cases of jargon dysphasia, comprehension loss cannot be regarded as the basic or even the most important symptom (Weinstein *et al.*, 1966). In jargon dysphasia there are commonly, moreover, a number of associated defects which are absent in pure word deafness, e.g. perseveration or over-abundance of speech.

Psychological mechanisms

Thanks to the work that was started in the field of communication engineering during the two World Wars, a good deal is known about the factors which affect auditory speech comprehension in normal people. This is not to say that we know how the process is carried out in the brain; only that we know some of the factors affecting it.

The three most important factors in the comprehension of language by normal people seem to be transitional probabilities, chunking and filtering.

Transitional probabilities. Because the number of different sounds available is smaller than the amount of information to be conveyed by them, and because the number of channels along which these sounds can be transmitted is limited, messages usually take the form of sound sequences, each sequence being a different signal. Thus we speak in words and in sentences rather than in single phonemes. But this habit of stringing sounds together in sequences, governed by grammatical and syntactical rules, means that most of what is said becomes redundant. If we have heard how the sequence starts we can more or less guess how it will end. The signals at the beginning of the sequence limit the range of the ones that can follow, so that we do not have to hear many of the words in a sentence to comprehend its meaning. We seem to have at our disposal a built-in computer working out the transitional probabilities of word strings which tells us which word to produce or expect at any moment. Our knowledge of a language depends on the extent to which this computer is programmed by past experience to carry out the operations.

Filtering. The importance of sound filtering in the comprehension process has mainly been studied by two-channel (dichotic) listening tasks. A subject listens through earphones to two simultaneous messages, one coming into his right ear and one to his left. He is asked to follow one of the messages only, and is able to do so by rejecting almost completely the sounds he hears in the other ('the cocktail party situation'). It is found that most of the rejected message is ignored completely, yet at the same time some aspects of it 'get through'. The subject can tell whether it is spoken by a man or a woman, in French or in English, fast or slowly: and if individual words in it have special emotional value or fit in well with the message being followed, the hearer will switch over to the rejected message and let it in (Treisman, 1965).

Chunking. It appears that one does not deal with the sounds individually in the exact order in which they are received. We seem to store them up in chunks and then decode the chunk as a whole rather than on the basis of its individual elements. Thus, when we hear the word 'butterfly' we do not think first of the word 'but', then reject this in favour of the word 'butter', and then reject both of those in favour of the whole word 'butterfly'. We seem to conceive the word 'butterfly' as a whole and right from the beginning. Recent work has shown that the amount that can be stored and decoded in a single chunk increases with age and experience. One of the chief characteristics of the speech-retarded child lies in the small amount that he can deal with in a given chunk.

In word deafness the use of transitional probabilities seems to be intact. The patients are still able to make use of contexts and, indeed, are even more reliant on them than before. It is in the spheres of chunking and filtering that the failure seems to lie.

Physiological mechanisms

A good deal of attention has been devoted to ascertaining the parts of the brain involved in understanding both speech and music. The difference between defects of musical and verbal comprehension arising from cerebral lesions has been studied systematically in patients with temporal lobe lesions by the psychologists at the Montreal Neurological Institute. Milner (1962) reported a selective deficit in tone discrimination (measured on the Seashore test) in patients with a dichotic listening task and at the same time found that patients with left temporal lesions made more errors than those with right ones in the repetition of digits. This latter deficit was further increased after left temporal lobectomy but was not influenced by right temporal lobectomy. Following this up Kimura (1964) compared patients with left and right temporal lobe lesions on dichotically presented melodies and digits, and confirmed the conclusion that melodies were more disturbed by right temporal lesions and digits by left.

Shankweiler (1966) further confirmed Kimura's finding in a careful study of twenty-one patients with left and twenty-four patients with right temporal lesions who showed no defect of hearing prior to the operation. Shankweiler and Harris (1966) found that, in their ability to recognize single consonants or vowels or even clusters of phonemes, dysphasic patients followed the normal pattern of behaviour; but in a further study of normal subjects on a dichotically presented series of synthetic speech sounds, Shankweiler and Studdert-Kennedy (1959) found that the difference between the right and left hemisphere lay in the identification of consonants only. Whereas vowels were recognized equally well by both ears, it was only on the recognition of consonants that the right ear was superior. This suggests that the right ear is selectively attuned to the recognition of 'on–off' stimuli, and that it is in the temporal sequencing of input that its supremacy lies. This finding confirms a suggestion of Efron (1963) who found that for two events to be judged as simultaneous, the one directed to the non-dominant hemisphere had to precede the other by 2 to 6 milliseconds. Efron suggests that signals reaching the non-dominant hemisphere have to be relayed to the dominant one, and that the matching or integration is carried out there. The study by Sparks and Geschwind (1968) of one patient with a surgically induced 'split brain' seems to add support to this suggestion, for their patient was totally unable to decode verbal signals applied to the left ear and hence only relayed to the right hemisphere.

When comparing the ability of patients with right- and left-hemisphere lesions to repeat sentences, Newcombe and Marshall (1967) found that the defect shown by the left-hemisphere patients was mainly seen on the semantic constraints. Grammatical constraints were not important. On this task patients with right-hemisphere lesions showed no deficit from normals, but Gazzaniga and Sperry (1967) do not agree that the right hemisphere is incapable of decoding speech sounds at all levels. In the three patients they studied after section of the cerebral commissures (i.e. the fibres connecting the two hemispheres), they found that the right hemisphere could recognize both object names and written material. The patients, for example, could pick out by feel or vision an object the name of which had been given to them in the left ear.

As with expression, speech comprehension seems to go with

handedness. Curry (1967) and Curry and Rutherford (1967) found that the better performance of the right over the left ear for the comprehension of dichotically presented words in normals was not so great in left handers as in right handers.

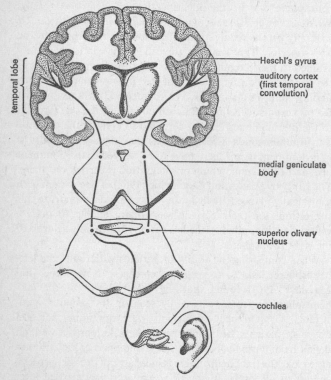

Figure 7 The auditory pathways and projections onto the temporal lobe

Of particular interest in this sphere are the observations made by Penfield and Perot (1963). Auditory experiences were often elicited by stimulation of the exposed superior first temporal convolution (see Figure 7) in patients undergoing craniotomy for the relief of epilepsy. Such phenomena were reported by 7·7 per cent of the 520 patients in whom the exposed temporal lobe was stimulated. 62·5 per cent of the experiences were reported by patients from stimulation of the non-dominant hemisphere. The experiences reported were usually the same as those experienced during the epileptic aura itself. While stimulation of the auditory sensory cortex (i.e. Heschl's gyrus, see Figure 7) only evoked buzzing, stimulation of the superior surface of the first temporal convolution evoked the same phenomena (voices, phrases or words) as were experienced during the epileptic aura.

Auditory plus visual experiences were also reported from twenty-two different points stimulated in thirteen patients. Thirteen of these points were again in the non-dominant hemisphere and only nine in the dominant hemisphere. Music was also experienced by eleven patients and more often again in the right than in the left superior temporal convolution. The authors dismissed the interpretation that this indicates the presence of 'engrams' in the temporal cortex itself by pointing out that stimulation of the area can still produce the experience even after the cortex has been removed. They do, however, suggest that this part of the cortex plays a part in the interpretation of sounds and renders the records of past experience available for this purpose.

Conclusions

While there seems ample evidence to indicate that disorders relating to vision are associated with lesions in the parieto-occipital lobe, those of the body image are associated with the parietal area, and those of audition with the temporal, there is still very little general agreement about what has actually gone wrong in those cases where it is disordered or how the normal processes of perception are mediated. We know that in normal perceptual processes, expectancy and set are of immense importance, and it is apparent that cerebral injury in no way diminishes this function. If anything, in fact, it increases it, for when the external stimuli which might negate an expectancy are reduced, the expectancy becomes belief. The patient truly believes that he sees, even though blind; he 'knows' his body to be intact even though half of it is paralysed. Thus, when immediate function is impaired there is a tendency for the functions developed over the past to be evoked again as if, once established, the function can carry on autonomously in the absence of the stimuli which originally aroused them. We know too that habits apparently suppressed or over-ruled by past experience are reawakened as if they were only dormant, lying ready in the background to take over once again. But, as Penfield points out, these observations do not prove that engrams subserving these habits are situated in the area whose derangement causes their release. Lesions in the temporo-parietal and occipital areas of the non-dominant hemisphere merely seem to reduce the amount of information reaching the subject which could be used to modify his expectancy, and this seems to be the probable basis of preceptual disorders.

How this reduction is brought about we still do not know for certain. Luria (see King, 1967) has suggested that injured parts of the brain cause a focus of excitation which inhibits the activity of the rest of the brain by negative induction. Birch, Belmont and Karp's (1967) experiments which indicated that injured brain areas are slower at processing sensory information than healthy ones supports this view; and the observation that in disorders of auditory perception the main defects lie in the quantity and speed of input which can be dealt with, is a further indication of it.

4 Disorders of Motor Skill and Verbal Expression

The disorders of skills which may follow cerebral lesions can be divided into those affecting motor power, those affecting the execution of the motor skills (apraxia) and those affecting speech (dysphasia) or reading and writing (dyslexia and dysgraphia). In this book, disorders due to loss of muscular power alone (paresis) will not be discussed. Nor will losses of skill due purely to poor motor control – ataxia, choreiform movements and tremors.

Apraxia

In true apraxia, the patient has little loss of power or control over his limbs but appears to have 'forgotten' how to carry out specific acts. When asked to touch his nose, he may touch instead the top of his head or his ears: when asked to comb his hair, he will turn the comb over and over in his hands two or three times or put it on the table; when asked to light a cigarette he will try to put the packet in his mouth and the cigarettes on the table. Such patients usually know what they are trying to do and recognize their inability to do it, shaking their head in perplexity and cursing their foolishness. Under emotional stress, or if the act is part of an automatic sequence, it may be completed adequately, but its execution is no longer under voluntary control. The harder the patient tries to carry it out and the more he concentrates on it, the more likely he is to fail.

Apraxias have been divided into ideomotor (the loss of skilled sequences), dressing (inability to dress) and constructional (inability to copy spatial configuration, build bricks and put things together).

Ideomotor apraxia

This term was coined by Liepmann in 1905 to indicate a disconnexion between the idea of a movement and ability to carry it out. Typical instances of ideomotor apraxia have just been described above. The disturbances are clearly recognized by both the patient and those looking after him, and need no special tests to elicit them. They refer to simple everyday tasks. Usually there is a relationship between the patient's ability to complete a task and the complexity of the task itself (the number of different isolated acts involved), and the frequency with which it has been performed; but the main defect always lies in the patient's inability to produce it at will. Thus a patient who is quite unable to take a match out of a box and light a candle put in front of her to command, may still be able to carry out these same acts if there were a sudden failure of the electricity. One who cannot put on her spectacles when the doctor asks her to may well do so in order to read. There are also frequently in such patients disorders of gesture and pantomine, such as those noted by Goodglass and Kaplan (1963) in a number of patients with dysphasia. Thus, if a patient is asked to show how he would stir sugar in a teacup, brush his teeth, etc. in the absence of the utensils, he would, like a small child, use some part of the body to indicate the utensil. Instead of holding an imaginary spoon to stir, he will stick a finger out and rotate it. Instead of holding an imaginary toothbrush, he will scratch the fore-finger over the teeth. Besides demonstrating the 'body-part as object' characteristic, these patients also tend to accompany their gestures with verbal commentaries (verbal overflow) and find the imitation of a gesture easier than its production from memory.

It is sometimes argued that two different forms of apraxia should be distinguished: motor apraxia (inability to carry out an act) and ideational apraxia (inability to plan it). Arguments for making this distinction are based on the observation that ability to demonstrate the use of objects (ideational apraxia) is only seen in lesions involving the left hemisphere, while the ability to make gestures (for example salute, wave, make a cross in the air and other motor aspects of behaviour) can occur in unilateral lesions in either hemisphere (de Renzi, Pieczuro and Vignolo, 1968).

Dressing apraxia

Inability on the part of the patient to dress himself is probably just one aspect of ideomotor apraxia, but as it is often the most obvious aspect and the one which attracts most attention, it has sometimes been described as an isolated symptom. As in ideomotor apraxia the patient does not lose the ability to put on his clothes, but only the ability to organize the sequence of acts necessary to do so. When trying to put on a coat, he cannot remember how to get his arm into the sleeve and ends up with it back to front. Tying bows and doing up buttons present particular difficulties, and it is in his attempts to carry out these acts that the patient suffering from apraxia is most easily distinguished from the one suffering from dementia, even though the end results are often the same in each case. Thus patients in both categories may finish up with their clothes on back to front, inside out, and upside down; they may try to pull their stockings on over their shoes or put on a coat before a shirt. Their reasons for doing so may be different in the two diagnostic categories, and further investigation is usually necessary before an ill-dressed patient can justifiably be said to demonstrate apraxia for dressing rather than neglect of one side of his body or a more generalized mental disorder.

Constructional apraxia

In contrast to the conditions described above wherein the patient shows inability to carry out skills that have been acquired and practised over a lifetime, constructional apraxia consists of the loss of the ability to apply practised skills to new situations – e.g. copy a design, draw a map of the ward, make a three-dimensional model with bricks. To elicit constructional apraxia, the patient must be faced with these tasks; hence while ideomotor and dressing apraxia are easily observable in a ward setting and are usually recognized by medical and nursing staff, the discovery and measurement of constructional apraxia is usually the prerogative of the psychologist with his battery of tests.

Tests commonly used to elicit constructional apraxia are described by Critchley (1953) and by Warrington (1969), and may be mentioned briefly here.

1. Paper and pencil tests. (a) Copying test: the subject is asked to copy designs of varying difficulty and complexity which involve at least two figures or lines in contact with one another, and some diagonals. (b) Drawing test: the patient is asked to draw a clock face, house, or a map.

2. Stick tests: the subject is presented with sticks of various lengths and is asked to copy a design made by the examiner. If he finds this too difficult, the task may be simplified by removing all those sticks except the ones essential for the task.

3. Brick building (three-dimensional) test: the subject is presented with a group of blocks of different shapes and sizes and asked to make them into a set of patterns (tower, bridge, etc.), or to copy patterns made by the examiner.

4. Block design: the subtest from the WAIS is a useful method of eliciting this defect. Subjects with constructional apraxia usually show undue difficulty with the very first of these designs, and break down on this test much earlier than would be expected from their performance on other subtests.

Scoring of constructional apraxia is most satisfactorily based on the presence of signs of abnormality and the difficulty (complexity) of the item eliciting them. The signs themselves have been well described by Critchley (1953) and by Warrington (1969). They are:

1. The copy cannot be placed in an appropriate place on the sheet of paper or the table. It may be started so close to one side that it must be pushed close together or fall off.

2. There is difficulty in bringing two lines or two designs together without overlapping, overshooting or remaining disconnected.

3. In line drawings the copy may be smaller or larger than the original.

4. There is a tendency to place vertical lines either too close together or too far apart. Single lines may be reduplicated.

5. The copy may be rotated in space (rotation) or placed on top of the original (crowding). In the stick and brick tests, the subject will remove parts of the original to make his own copy, and has difficulty in selecting those of the right size or length.

6. Sections may be omitted without the subject apparently noticing it. This is particularly common if visuo-spatial agnosia is also present, for then the patient tends to include in his reproductions only the right side of the model or the object that he is attempting to draw, omitting the left. If asked to place the numbers on a clock face, or the hand at a certain time, the numbers will be crowded together on the right or written underneath one another in a column. The big and little hands may be confused or placed on top of one another.

Psychological and physiological mechanisms

The mechanism responsible for these disorders has been discussed to some extent in recent literature, and since most of the conclusions are based on the different patterns of breakdown associated with different locations of lesions, it seems logical to consider the physiological and psychological hypotheses together in this section. There is fairly conclusive evidence that apraxia is only seen in connexion with lesions in the parietal area (see Figure 5, p. 70), and a further distinction can be drawn between those associated with left-, those associated with right- and those associated with bilateral hemisphere lesions. Warrington (1969) has further analysed the different ways in which constructional apraxia manifests itself in right- or left-hemisphere lesions under three headings: (a) the incidence and severity of the disability, (b) the qualitative differences and (c) associated disabilities.

The incidence of constructional apraxia appears to be almost twice as common after right- as after left-sided lesions but this is closely related to associated disabilities, notably slow reaction time, unilateral neglect and loss of topographical memory, all of which occur more often after right- than after left-hemisphere lesions. Many authors have argued that inability to carry out constructional tasks may be due to these associated disabilities rather than to any direct interference with the skill. Indeed analysis of the errors made by right- as opposed to left-hemisphere lesion patients supports this conclusion to some extent. Patients with right-sided lesions tend to copy designs in a fragmented and disjointed manner whereas those with left-sided lesions simplify them and can only succeed at all by 'slavishly reproducing the lines'. The right-sided patients include all the details but often in their wrong places: the left-sided patients miss the details out. Attempts to quantify these differences has proved extremely hard.

Although it is not truly an apraxic condition, Gazzaniga, Bogan and Sperry (1965) have described a remarkable disconnexion between motor responses and the stimuli arousing them in patients subjected to section of the corpus callosum (Figure 8). Thus, if asked to pick up objects corresponding to visual stimuli presented in one half field, such patients can only respond appropriately with the hand controlled by the hemisphere receiving the visual impressions – the right hand can pick out objects corresponding to images in the right visual field and the left hand can match those in the left, but cross-hemisphere matching is not accomplished beyond the chance expectation. The possible anatomical basis for this is discussed at length by Geschwind (1965).

The association between dysphasia and apraxia will be discussed in more detail later. In the meantime it may be noted that while the lesions associated with apraxic conditions are predominantly bilateral, those affecting speech are predominantly unilateral.

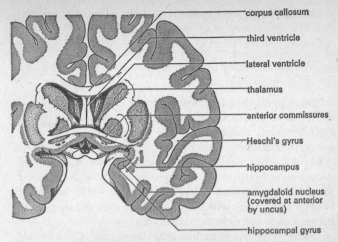

corpus callosum

third ventricle

lateral ventricle

thalamus

anterior commissures

Heschl's gyrus

hippocampus

amygdaloid nucleus
(covered at anterior
by uncus)

hippocampal gyrus

Figure 8 Transverse section of the brain through the anterior
commissures

Disorders of Verbal Expression

Disorders of speech (dysphasia or aphasia) are a common
sequel to cerebral injury and have been noted for many years.
The most obvious impairment refers to the naming of objects.
Rochford (1969) in a short history of aphasiology, writes:

An early example was a case described by Napoleon's surgeon
Baron Leary. In the Battle of Waterloo a soldier received a 'wound
of the brain' after which his intellect was said to be impaired and he
could not remember proper names or substantives. He returned to
work as a drill sergeant but found himself unable to teach 'naming
of parts' without consulting the manual, nor could he call his men
by name.

However, this loss of the ability to name objects (anomia, nominal
aphasia or amnesic aphasia) is not always associated with the
inability to find nouns – only inability to associate them with the
objects to which they usually refer. Bateman (in 1890) quotes a case
of Trousseau's who said 'pig, brute, stupid fool' to a visitor pointing
to a chair, and one could not say that such an outburst involved
inability to find nouns even though there is clearly a lack of naming

as such. Moreover, it is frequently noted that patients who may not be able to find a name at the moment it is requested can find it in another context. 'But Doctor, I can't say no', exclaimed a patient of Hughlings Jackson. Thus as Schuell and Brown (in 1950) point out, the disorder refers to the inability to find words as required, not just to name objects.

Speech is disturbed in psychiatric patients as well as those with focal cerebral lesions, but in general the psychotic speech disorders can be distinguished from those due to focal cerebral lesions by the following points:

1. Adults with speech disturbances of organic origin are seldom completely dumb. Unlike some psychotic patients the dysphasic patient usually has a number of words or sounds left in his repertoire which he may repeat over and over again but seldom in the right context.

2. The dysphasic patient nearly always tries hard to communicate and usually succeeds in doing so, whereas in the psychotic patient (senile as well as schizophrenic), communication seems to be irrelevant.

The way and degree to which practical language is impaired by focal cerebral lesions varies between individuals and in the same individual at different times. In some, expression may be limited as mentioned above to a few single words or stock phrases (standard aphasia – see Weinstein and Keller, 1963). In others fluency and normal word sequencing are retained (in fact may even be over-abundant) but the words uttered do not make sense (neologisms) and the sentences are meaningless (jargon aphasia). In yet others it is not so much the knowledge of the words but the ability to articulate them which is absent (verbal aphasia).

Standard aphasia

Although the inability to find names as required may predominate over the ability to string words together in sentences (agrammatism), and vice versa, it is now generally agreed that the disorders of speech arising from cerebral injury in standard aphasia are difficult to place in separate categories and especially to associate with different cerebral lesions. Head (1926) regarded the ability to find names as an important symptom, and referred to at least three cases in which it was the sole residual symptom; but even he, when classifying the speech disorders into separate categories, stressed that each of his groups included disorders of wider extent. Weisenberg and McBride (1935) regarded dysphasia as classifiable only into expressive and receptive disorders. This conclusion is also reached by Rochford and Williams (1964) who studied thirty-three consecutive patients admitted to the neurosurgical wards at Oxford with organic speech disorders on a battery of tests measuring naming, the comprehension of names, reading and writing, all of which were equated for difficulty and scored in terms of age equivalents based on the performance of children between five and eleven years. They found only three patients out of the thirty-three who showed impairment on the object-naming test as a sole symptom. If naming of objects was severely impaired in their patients, there was also gross impairment on all other tests. Comprehension of names was, however, unimpaired in twenty of the patients who showed disorders in other spheres. Impairment in the visual aspects of language (reading and writing) was closely correlated ($r = +0.74$), and was the sole language impairment in two cases, suggesting that this aspect of language occurs as a separate disorder.

Investigating their patients further, Rochford and Williams found that the inability to name objects was paralleled by the inability to name actions (verbs) and colours. Thus, the naming of objects is probably not an isolated disability. Nevertheless, it is a task which is easily studied, open to experimental manipulation and can be controlled. Using it as a basis for their main investigation, Rochford and Williams (1962, 1963, 1965) tried to define some of the factors involved in the word finding of dysphasic patients, and to relate these to the linguistic processes of normal individuals. By comparing dysphasic patients with those suffering from senile dementia, they were able to show that dysphasia is independent of memory, perception, intellectual deficit and fatigue, since although these factors all influenced the performance of senile patients, they did not affect the performance of the dysphasic ones.

Factors involved in standard aphasia

Frequency. Turning to the variables within language itself which influence word finding, one of the easiest to study is frequency, i.e. the relative number of times a word is spoken. The most accurate information available concerning the frequency of word usage is the Thorndike and Lorge Word Count (Thorndike and Lorge, 1944), column G of which was compiled in 1944 from a comprehensive sample of written language. This word count uses the following notation: A.A. indicates words occurring more than 100 times per million words; A. indicates words occurring between fifty and 100 times per million. Other words are given a number indicating the number of occurrences per million words.

In the studies of Rochford and Williams, eighteen objects were drawn in simple outline each on a plain white card. The names for these objects ranged from words occurring 100 times or over, or between fifty and 100 times per million (A.A. or A. words) to words occurring only eight times per million. They were all common objects which normal adults can name without difficulty and which have one unequivocal name in the English language.

There was a close correlation ($r = +0.79$) between the word frequency of an item and the number of errors made by dysphasic patients. There was still a positive but smaller ($r = +0.34$) correlation in the senile patients whose performance was very variable. Word frequency was also seen to affect the ease with which items other than common objects were named. Thus the names for actions (verbs), colours and even body parts have varied word frequency. In each of these tests a relationship was found between errors and word frequency in the dysphasic patients.

Sequencing. Once a single word or name is found, those that 'go with' or follow it in practice seem to be aroused automatically. The English language contains many composite nouns which are largely descriptive of the objects they name – e.g. 'wheelbarrow'. These composite words can be divided into four groups depending on the word frequency of the different syllables: common–rare (e.g. 'sundial', 'pennyfarthing', 'hedgehog'), common–common ('lighthouse', 'penknife', 'horseshoe'), rare–common ('spinningwheel', 'padlóck'), and rare–rare. The proportion of errors made by dysphasic patients when asked to name such objects depends on the frequency of the first syllable only. If this is common, the whole word is easy to find; if it is rare, the word is difficult to find.

Context. Patients are often able to find words in their common verbal contexts when not able to do so without a context at all. A group of dysphasic patients was asked to name a number of objects and for each one that they failed to name they were offered a variety of cues or prompts. One of these was a verbal sentence in which the word sought would normally be the last item. Thus for the word 'hand' the cue was 'We have feet and —', for the word 'teeth' 'We bite with our —'. This cue was found to be effective in eliciting the word required in many cases (Rochford and Williams, 1963).

The situation in which a word is being sought and the frequency with which it has been used before in *that situation*, is another factor found to be important. There are many words in the English language which are used in a number of different contexts and denote completely different things in each one. For example, the word 'bat' refers to a cricket bat or a flying mouse. Dysphasic patients are able to find the word in its common context (as deduced from the Thorndike–Lorge Semantic Word Count, 1938) more easily than in its rare one.

Arousal of phonetic elements. It is seen from the above two investigations that sequencing and context both appear to give dysphasic subjects a lead-in to the required word and so help them to find it. Does arousal of the phonetic elements of the word itself help?

1. *Arousal by rhymes*. In the prompting investigation described under 'Context', one of the prompts used was a rhyme to the required word. Thus for the word 'hand' they were told 'it rhymes with band'. These cues were found by Rochford and Williams to have no significant effect on the dysphasic patient's ability to find words; in fact, in not a single instance was a word found in response to this cue alone. This point will be discussed again when we come to consider the relation between dysphasic disorders and normal speech. The generalization of words on the basis of rhyming patterns seems to be a phase through which normal children pass between the ages of five to ten, but thereafter dies out (Rochford and Williams, 1963).

2. *Arousal of the word in a different context*. If a word is aroused in one situation or by one means it is thereafter found more easily in another. Thus, once the word had been found in its common usage in the task described in the section on 'Context' it could then, more often than not, be applied to its rare one. 'Of course, those are the teeth too.'

3. *Arousal by spelling*. Finally, a cue well known to be very affective is that of beginning to spell out the word sought, 'It begins with H,' 'It's an H A N –.'

From the above investigation it becomes clear that the word store of dysphasic patients is not so much destroyed as relatively inaccessible. Access to individual items can be gained either by some form of lead-in (semantic or contextual) or by arousal of the required item which immediately lowers its threshold to reproduction (de-blocking – Weigl, 1963). The effectiveness of the letters used to spell the word in writing suggests that words are coded in their written and spoken forms close together. However, it must be remembered that rhymes did not assist production. Perhaps the failure of a rhyme is due to the fact that it arouses only the last sound of a word, not its beginning, whereas the first letter of a word arouses its beginning rather than its end. The relative effectiveness of the first syllable of a composite word (as against that of the last syllable) also indicates that it is the initial lead-in to the word that is the difficulty for the dysphasic patient, not its production once it has been, so to speak, located. The same is certainly true for normal people. Any crossword puzzle enthusiast will have realized that the assistance given by the first letter of a missing word is infinitely greater than that given by the last.

Consistency

It has often been claimed that the speech of dysphasic patients is so fluctuating and inconsistent that any attempt to assess it in quantitative terms is doomed to failure. However, if the conditions under which dysphasic patients are asked to produce words are truly held constant, their performance becomes remarkably stable. Thus, the variability so often described in the accounts of dysphasia may be due to the variable conditions under which it was examined.

Although the systematic investigations reported here have been carried out on single words – indeed, most of them are on single object names – it must be mentioned again that in general conversation and in many practical situations, some dysphasic patients appear to have less difficulty in finding single words than they do in stringing words together in sequences, or putting them in their right grammatical form. The suffixes denoting past and present tenses are confused; that denoting an adverb (-ly) is added or subtracted to a verb indiscriminately.

Unfortunately systematic study of these disorders and the conditions associated with them have not yet been carried out with adult dysphasic patients.

Jargon aphasia

Quite different from standard aphasia and characterized by its poor communication value and its over-abundance of output, jargon aphasia has been recognized as a separate category of speech disorder from standard aphasia by most observers. An example of one man attempting to describe the 'telegraph boy' picture from the Terman Merrill Test (Figure 9) is given below.

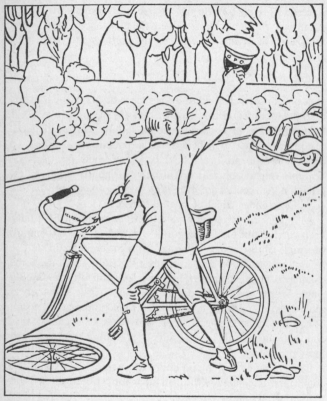

Figure 9

The telephone man in the process of describing the existence and spectatorship of . . . in the West Country (yes). The tunnership here . . . the form utterige of the er vessel, it really is what's in its front tyre plus not, are you with me? (no – would you explain). In order to find the tyreship there you'd run the tyre into the front wheel and then you'd weigh it, and then you'd have the weight of the front tyre, er it may be there's no great problem there as far as I see it. The, the, the, the cycle tube for the front tyre hasn't had a bad break down, isn't going to have one and it can't have one anyway, so your piterist is quite all right (Rochford, 1969).

The verbal output of such patients has been described by Valpeau in 1843 (see Rochford, 1969) as 'intolerable loquacity' by Freud (1891) as 'impoverishment of words with abundance of speech impulse' and by Jackson (1866) as 'peculiar and outwardly meaningless language form'. As with standard aphasia many attempts have been made to attribute the disorders to some function other than the linguistic one, but nearly all can be refuted. Impoverishment of general intellectual ability and visual perceptual disorders were not found in the two cases of jargon aphasia described by Kinsbourne and Warrington (1963c), and although memory is difficult to assess in these patients, and may indeed be poor, there is no certain evidence that it is.

Weinstein et al. (1966) attribute jargon to lack of self-awareness (monitoring) or anosognosia, but Kinsbourne and Warrington and Rochford believe that jargon aphasics are able to understand their own output if this is played back to them after very short time intervals, and occasionally they show some insight into their errors. Although the comprehension of others may be impaired, it is certainly not totally absent, and is usually much better preserved than in patients with word deafness. Thus the tendency to talk jargon cannot be *due* to comprehension loss.

Factors within the speech of jargon aphasia itself have been studied by Weinstein et al. (1966) and by Rochford (1969). Rochford described four cases; one, a traumatic aphasic, was seen on five different occasions during the three months he took to recover, another was seen on three different occasions during the course of recovery. The points noted by Rochford were:

1. There was a close relationship between the total number

of errors made on a naming test and the total number of words emitted during the course of it. (See Figure 10.)

2. There was less correspondence between word frequency and errors in these patients than in standard aphasics.

3. There was often an associative relationship between the words that were uttered and the words that were sought, even though this could not always be recognized immediately.

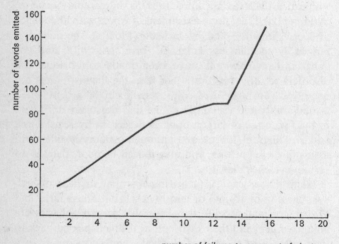

Figure 10 The relationship between the number of words emitted and total number of errors on a naming test for jargon aphasics

4. There was considerably more perseveration in patients with jargon aphasia than in those with standard aphasia, and the perseverative disturbances spread over a longer time interval.

5. The speech of jargon aphasics was similar in certain respects to that of psychotic patients. Thus jargon aphasics, like schizophrenic patients, often refer to themselves in the third person, use many personal references and often resort to original metaphor.

6. Although flashes of insight may be apparent occasionally,

it is much more common for the patient to appear unaware of his mistake. Thus one patient, described by Rochford, when asked if he had any difficulty finding words, replied: 'No, none at all. I come out of my speech making to everything like that, quite quite comfortably, thank you.'

In their interpretation of jargon aphasia, both Weinstein and Rochford stress the failure of monitoring: whether failure is due to the fact that too much output is presented for adequate filtering or whether it is inadequate filtering that allows the excessive output, is impossible to say. Kinsbourne and Warrington believe the speech of the jargon 'approximates quite closely to the patient's uncorrected and unexpurgated inner speech'; Rochford's conclusions are somewhat similar. Rochford points out that a characteristic of most patients with organic cerebral involvement – and clearly shown in his own cases – is inability to give word associations as required. Thus, when one of Rochford's patients was still trying to name every object shown to him with a flood of associative answers, he was reduced to almost complete dumbness when specifically asked to *give* associations to the same words. This paradox – and the distinction between standard and jargon aphasia – is explained by Rochford in the following way. In standard aphasia the threshold of all items in the word store is raised so that, in order to find any one at any time, excessive stimulation is required. In jargon aphasia the threshold is lowered so that all are aroused and the difficulty lies in sorting out the appropriate item from the mass of words presenting themselves. The direction of 'spread' in both cases follows normal associational patterns. Thus, according to Rochford, 'the jargon dysphasic's inability to name does not lie behind his verbal excitement, but is the result of it.'

Verbal apraxia

Defects of articulation can vary from a simple slurring of consonants (dysarthria) or a change of melodic tone (dysprosody) to complete inability to organize the articulatory mechanism for the production of words (aphasia). Often some defects of word finding may accompany these disorders, but in several cases, some with clearly localized lesions (Whitty, 1964), apraxia of the articulatory mechanism can occur as an isolated symptom.

Although this type of dysphasia has been recognized for a long time, it seems to have been less systematically studied than the others, and has not received any special attention from psychologists.

Dysphasia in childhood

The disorders of language shown by children who suffer brain damage of the dominant hemisphere are different from those of adults in that:

1. Residual speech is much rarer and seldom contains the paraphasias, stereotopies and perseverations seen in adults.

2. Reading and writing is nearly always severely impaired alongside any loss of expression.

3. Articulatory disturbances are commonly seen alongside loss of word finding.

Thus the brain-damaged child tends to remain mute or to emit only the simplest, most automatic phrases when questioned, saying most of the time 'I don't know' or 'I can't'.

Alajouanine and L'Hermitte (1965) noted that this gross loss of speech tends to be replaced by the adult type of dysphasia as the age at which trauma is sustained increases. The speed of recovery, however, shows an inverse relationship with age – the younger the child at the age of trauma, the quicker and more complete is its recovery.

Relationship between dysphasia and normal speech processes

Although standard dysphasia renders its sufferers unable to retrieve or find access to words, the rules which govern dysphasic speech production are the same as in normal people (Howes and Geschwind, 1961). Moreover, if the intellectual activity or alertness of normal people is temporarily reduced, they are found to show many of the features common to dysphasia. For example, it is well known that alcoholic intoxication produces slurring of speech (dysarthria) together with a loquacity comparable in some ways to jargon aphasia. ECT reduces the naming ability of patients in exactly the same way as dysphasia, access to the lower frequency words being the last to be regained (Rochford and Williams, 1962). Distraction on a dichotic listening task not only reduces word finding (again the loss is relative to word frequency) but the errors made by normal people under these conditions are closely related to the errors made by dysphasics (Rochford and Williams, 1962). Finally, Oldfield and Wingfield (1965) have found the same parallel occurring between word frequency and naming latency in normal people as occurs between word frequency and naming ability in dysphasia: the rare words taking longer to find by normal subjects just as they are less likely to be found by the dysphasic patients.

These findings all indicate that the loss of word finding in standard dysphasia represents an exaggeration of a condition common to all linguistic expression. By focusing attention on some of the factors and conditions influencing dysphasia, the study of brain-damaged patients has also drawn attention to some of these factors in the normal subject – particularly the effects of frequency and of sequence constraints. But it has not only told us something about how the mechanism (often likened to a computer) works; it has also told us a little about how it comes to be established or programmed.

This is not the place to discuss the development of language in children – a subject to which much attention is being currently paid and of which several reviews have been published – but it may be noted in passing that the pattern of breakdown in dysphasic children does indicate that the mechanisms used by adults to find and produce words develop only slowly over the course of time. The dysphasia shown by children also tells us that the skills least practised are those first to go. The close parallel between the age at which words are learned by children and the difficulty with which they are found by dysphasic adults (Rochford and Williams, 1962) is another indication of the relationship between development and breakdown. To assume, however, that brain damage causes simple regression would be dangerous. Both development and breakdown are dependent on certain factors, one of these clearly being frequency of usage.

It has been pointed out above that language depends on (a) the presence of a store of words, (b) the ability to select any item from this store at a single moment in time (retrieval) and (c) the emission of words in strings or sequences (syntax). We still do not know where and how the items in the vocabulary are stored or the connexion between this store and cerebral activity in general. We do know, however, that the items are stored in groups rather than as individuals (the arousal of one member of a group arouses others too); that a single item (e.g. the word 'hands') is stored several times over for each of its contexts, but that there is some relationship between these independent stores, since arousal of a word in one context can arouse it in others too. We also know that the written and spoken forms of a word are stored separately and yet with connexions between them.

We know, too, that with increasing age the groupings made between words is based on semantic rather than phonetic similarity although in the early stages of development this may not be so.

Physiological basis of dysphasia

That disorders of language are closely associated with injury to the dominant cerebral hemisphere is now well established. Within this area, further specialization seems to occur. While Broca's area (see Figure 11) is concerned mainly with articulation, word-finding difficulty is more often seen after lesions in the temporal lobe.

But because lesions in clearly defined areas cause clearly defined disorders it does not follow that the language function is necessarily stored in those areas. Indeed, language can still be emitted to some extent even after complete obliteration of the left hemisphere in a right-handed person. Smith (1966b) describes a forty-seven-year-old, right-handed man in whom the whole of the left hemisphere was removed for the treatment of a neoplastic lesion but who, six months after operation, was able to comprehend all that was said to him and was even able to utter short, simple stereotyped phrases, obey written as well as spoken commands and sing tunes to command. This suggests that even if verbal expression is confined to the activity of the left hemisphere comprehension of speech is not; and Jackson's contention that whereas propositional speech

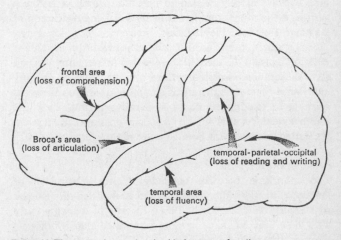

frontal area
(loss of comprehension)

Broca's area
(loss of articulation)

temporal-parietal-occipital
(loss of reading and writing)

temporal area
(loss of fluency)

Figure 11 The cortical areas involved in language functions

may be confined to the dominant hemisphere, emotive speech can be carried out by the other, is confirmed. However, a clear understanding of the role played by the right hemisphere in speech is difficult to obtain for, as Archibald and Wepman (1968) point out, in most cases of right-hemisphere injury other factors such as perseveration and general intellectual deterioration make the assessment of the language function extremely difficult. This is also the view of Serafetinides and Falconer (1963) after a study of the speech disorders associated with temporal lobe seizures.

Recovery of speech

The degree to which language functions show improvement during the course of time (even when the lesion itself is irreversible) raises many questions. Has the function been taken over by other cerebral areas, or is language itself really mediated by some other source? There seems to be little doubt that recovery from dysphasia and adequacy in the use of language are closely related to age. The earlier a lesion is sustained the more complete is likely to be the restitution of language function. Nevertheless, recovery can proceed surprisingly far in adults even if it does not begin immediately. Blakemore and Falconer (1967) followed up patients who had received left temporal lobectomies for the relief of epilepsy and found that while there was a considerable drop in verbal learning in the immediate post-operative period, and little improvement on this in the first two post-operative years, thereafter improvement became quite rapid.

Speech and handedness

The connexion between handedness and localization of language has been discussed and debated at length (Russell and Espir, 1961; Zangwill, 1963). In general it seems fairly clear now that language is more often mediated by the left than by the right hemisphere, in left-handed as well as in right-handed subjects, but that left-handed people will be less severely dysphasic than right-handed ones after left temporal lobe lesions, and will recover more quickly. Thus in left-handed subjects it is surmised that language is more evenly represented throughout both hemispheres than it is in strongly right-handed ones, but that even in them there is a predilection for representation in the left cerebral hemisphere. Further evidence, that in right-handers language is the prerogative of one hemisphere only, comes from the work of Gazzaniga and Sperry (1967) on patients in whom the cerebral commisures had been sectioned. It was found that following the operation, in which the two hemispheres of the brain were completely separated, visual stimuli presented in the right visual field (and therefore entering the left hemisphere) were named and described without difficulty, although those presented to the left and, therefore, decoded in the right hemisphere evoked 'only irrelevant confabulatory spoken responses or none at all'.

The possibility that language is affected by subcortical as well as by cortical lesions has often been raised, and there is some evidence – derived from the operations that were performed for the relief of Parkinsonian symptoms (wherein

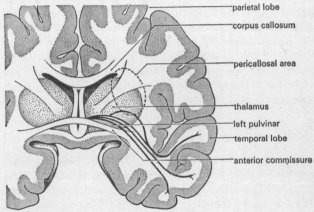

Figure 12 The subcortical areas involved in language functions

electrodes are stereotactically inserted in the area around the basal ganglia) – that this is indeed the case. Ojemann, Fedio and Van Buren (1968) found that stimulation of the left pulvinar and deep parietal white substance in the pericallosal region of both hemispheres through implanted electrodes, caused temporary inability to find names, even though automatic speech and consciousness were unaffected. (See Figure 12.)

In summary, it seems clear that even though the left temporal region may not be the only cerebral area involved in verbal expression or the only area capable of mediating it, this is the area used by normal people. This is not to say that language is localized within it. We walk with our legs, but walking is not a special faculty localized within the legs. In the same way we name objects, i.e. we make certain phonetic and articulatory acts when confronted with them – we do not possess a special faculty for naming. Instead of speaking of a word store and its organization, our thinking might be more precise if we confined ourselves to a description of the acts. Walking is the name given to one of the functions performed by the legs – a function which, if the legs are injured or amputated, can still be carried out, even though less efficiently, by muscle groups attached to the trunk. If linguistic expression is regarded in the same way it must be concluded that, while the function is normally carried out by the left hemisphere, when this is absent or injured at an early age other cerebral areas may take over the function using different strategies.

Dyslexia and Dysgraphia

Since disturbances of reading (dyslexia) and writing (dysgraphia) are often seen in the same subject and at the same time, it seems reasonable to consider them together. This does not mean to say that they are a single function. Indeed not only do they sometimes break down independently of one another, but both reading and writing may each be disturbed for a number of different reasons.

The disorders of reading seen after cerebral injury can be divided into those of visual and those of verbal origin.

Dyslexia – *visual origin*

Many disorders seem to stem from purely perceptual disturbances and would have been considered in the previous chapter had it not seemed more logical to deal with them here. Thus one patient may have difficulty fixating the stimuli and so miss out part of each word or sentence (Kinsbourne and

Warrington, 1962). Another may have difficulty in following sequences from left to right, so tending to see words in a haphazard way. Yet a third may be unable to recognize the visual aspects of letters or words but will be able to do so if he can move his hands over raised written material. Sometimes the perceptual difficulty can lead to writing errors. For example, a subject who can spell words orally without difficulty may be unable to do so in writing because the visual impression of what he puts on to the paper confuses him. He will stop half-way through a word, unable to see which letters he has already written and repeat some again. He will miss out letters thinking he has already put them in.

The disorders mentioned above are not very often seen in the discrete form described above. Far more frequently they are combined with difficulties in associating the visual forms of words or letters with their counterparts as will be described below.

Dyslexia – verbal origin

In these cases the difficulty lies not in recognizing the visual stimuli but in matching them to their appropriate verbal output. Thus written words can be matched to objects but not read aloud; or if the subject tries to enunciate them he may make the same paraphasic errors as he would in naming objects. Newcombe and Marshall (1966) describe one patient who read the word 'antique' as 'vase', 'canary' as 'parrot', 'gnome' as 'pixie', and the sentence 'put five shillings on a good horse' as 'five bob best horse'. Letters may be even harder to name than words, but in the case of the latter there is a close parallel between the words which children find hard to read (as judged by the age at which they are learned) and breakdown after cerebral injury. Thus reading ability after cerebral damage, like expression, can usefully be assessed on an age-equivalent scale (Rochford and Williams, 1964).

Dysgraphia

The disturbances of writing seen after cerebral injury can be divided into motor and ideational. The *motor* defects consist of (a) inability to put the letters of a word or the words of a sentence correctly in space (i.e. the lines become confused, run off the page, etc.), (b) perseveration (i.e. reduplication) of some letters (particularly those with loops, 'l's, 'm's, 'n's) and (c) reversals ('p' for 'b'). The basic disorder here is one of praxis, not of linguistics, and the same sort of mistakes are made as in drawing, building bricks, etc.

The *ideational* defects are concerned mostly with spelling. 'I can't remember how it goes,' a subject will remark. Kinsbourne and Warrington (1964) believe that a large proportion of the spelling mistakes seen in dysgraphia can be divided into two groups: those in which letters are added or omitted and those in which letter order is incorrect. While the former reflect 'an underlying disorder of language function' the latter reflect a more general difficulty in processing information in terms of spatiotemporal sequence.

Relation between dyslexia, dysgraphia and other disorders of language

As has already been mentioned, disorders of reading and writing may be seen in the absence of other linguistic disturbances. Where this is so they are predominantly of the sensory or motor type and do not involve impairment of the language function itself. Nevertheless, in the majority of instances dyslexia and dygraphia *are* associated with dysphasia and do involve much more than loss of reading and writing alone. Thus out of thirty-two dysphasic patients studied by Rochford (1969), twenty-one showed impairment of reading and writing. There were only four patients who showed defects in reading and writing with intact expression, and seven who showed a discrepancy in the opposite direction. Again in children, as has already been mentioned, language impairment is almost always associated with marked loss of reading and writing, relative to the degree to which those skills have been practised.

Nevertheless, two points are worth noting:

1. If the disorders of reading and writing are relatively more severe than the disorders in other language functions it is

probable that a lesion is localized in the parieto-occipital area (see Figure 13).

2. The defects in reading following cerebral lesions relate more to the execution than to the understanding of the word, just as the loss of speech relates to expression more than to comprehension. Thus as will be seen from Figure 13 patients with temporal or parietal lobe lesions are usually better able to match words to pictures or objects than to read the words aloud. This contrasts markedly with the performance of patients whose speech disorders are accompanied by dementia or psychotic illnesses in whom the opposite occurs and who may respond to the printed stimulus with the appropriate linguistic output, even though they seem to have little idea to what the word refers.

Dyslexia and the development of reading

What relation does acquired dysphasia and dysgraphia have to reading backwardness in children, and specifically to the conditions sometimes known as congenital dyslexia or word blindness? Backwardness in learning to read can have a number of different causes including low I.Q., poor visual discrimination, language disorder, educational insufficiency and emotional disturbances (Vernon, 1957). When all these factors have been discounted, however, there still remains a small group of children who seem incapable of learning to read and write, and in whom a variety of other features are nearly always found. These children may have difficulty in scanning systematically from left to right; they are often left-handed (or come from predominantly left-handed families) and tend to write from right to left instead of from left to right thus strengthening their scanning defects. They also frequently have poor visual imagery. Many of these children are known to have suffered some form of birth injury or were premature babies, and several show features of Gerstmann's syndrome including finger agnosia and right–left disorientation. According to Vernon, they 'belong to a class possessing

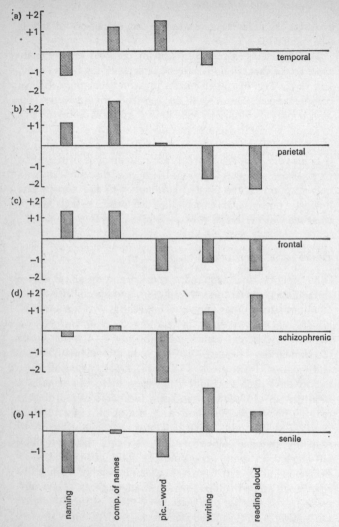

Figure 13 The relationship between performances of schizophrenic and senile patients and those with temporal, parietal or frontal lobe lesions on such tasks as reading aloud or picture–word matching (reproduced from *Speech Pathology and Therapy*, vol. 7, 1963)

a congenital disposition towards a set of defects of which reading disability is one.'

Together with their inability to read, their writing is usually abysmal. Miles (1967) gives the following example:

Mary I.Q. 131. Age 10·1
Wlter rolgh was a yound menn m woust to rob sponsch treasure shreps and he was a grote fo (crossed out) fat (crossed out and 't' altered to 'v') fovout af the Quen and he bunnt the fleat of sbne in the horber and he co (crossed out) cone book and said he had bur the kens of spoin bred.

A parallel between the defects shown by such children and those shown by patients suffering from traumatic dyslexia or dysgraphia is clear; but whereas in the latter cerebral pathology is almost always evident, there is as yet no conclusive evidence of an organic basis for the congenital defects.

Psychological mechanisms

Although the defects seen in children cannot be tied down to a definite organic cause, the studies carried out on them have given us some insight into the psychological mechanisms on which reading and writing depend. Systematic visual scanning from side to side (left to right in European and Arabic languages, right to left in Hebrew) seems to be an essential for reading and to some extent for writing, and where this is absent, either for congenital or traumatic reasons, the attainment or execution of these skills is impaired.

At the same time association between visual and verbal systems must also be made. Phonetic elements and visual signals must be closely associated, as indeed they are in normal subjects (Conrad, 1964). Inability to make this association may be one of the bases for congenital dyslexia as well as for the acquired reading and writing disorders, and is one of the symptoms nearly always present in organic dyslexia and dysgraphia.

Acalculia, or inability to carry out calculations, often accompanies loss of reading and writing and is commonly associated with Gerstmann's syndrome, but is occasionally the outstanding symptom of cerebral dysfunction. Gloning, Gloning and Hoff (1968) argue that disturbances of this skill are related more closely to the strategies a patient uses for calculation (whether he is a visualizer or a verbalizer) than to the site and nature of the lesion causing it.

Calculating, like reading, depends on a great many integrated functions – recognizing figures, remembering the tables, ordering numbers in rows and columns, etc. It is clear that a disorder which affects any of these functions will also affect a person's ability to calculate. However, it must be noted that patients who have lost the ability to recognize words or letters may still, on occasion, be able to recognize numerals, and vice versa.

Physiological mechanisms

In searching for a physiological basis for dyslexia, dysgraphia and acalculia it must be recognized that at least four functions are involved: the ability to control eye movements, the ability to co-ordinate these with hand movements, the ability to associate both these to words and, finally, the ability to understand what the words or letters mean.

The data support a supposition that each of these functions is closely associated with a different cerebral area. The purely visual or motor disorders are most often impaired in lesions in the parietal lobes; the association between these and the motor processes of execution are disturbed by parietotemporal lesions and the ability to give meaning to the symbols is disturbed by frontal lesions. Moreover, the disorders associated with congenital dyslexia or word blindness all suggest that functional impairment of the dominant parietal lobe is present in children showing this condition, and thus further emphasizes the necessity for this area in the acquisition of the skills involved.

However, although these cerebral areas may be (and, if present, apparently are) used for the specific functions listed, they are obviously not essential, for children in whom the entire left hemisphere is injured at birth (or removed for the relief of epilepsy) can still learn to read and write adequately and may attain almost normal standards in these skills. That experience at an optimal period causes specialization of these areas seems, however, to be indubitable. Although some function may be mediated by subcortical areas, the skills demonstrated are at a very elementary level.

Conclusions

At the end of the last chapter, it was suggested that the defects of perception arising from cerebral lesions are due to the fact that modes of reaction established from previous experience persist in an inappropriate form when modifying influences from the present external environment fail to reach them. In this chapter we have dealt with the breakdown of the reaction patterns themselves. It has been stressed that the individual acts are not so severely involved as the ability to integrate them into meaningful or useful sequences. A match can be held between the finger but cannot be struck on the side of the matchbox and held to the tip of a cigarette. A word can be uttered but not in the appropriate circumstances.

It has also been stressed that although verbal and manual skills are closely interconnected, the two hemispheres of the brain seem to be differentiated in the extent to which they control performance. It has also been stressed, however, that the acts performed, the end-product of these cerebral processes are, and must always be regarded merely as, acts: they do not have reality except when they are being performed. Hence to try and localize them in any structure is as meaningless as trying to localize 80 m.p.h. in one particular car. Why and when the acts are performed depends not only on the external situation but also to some extent on factors to be considered in the next chapter.

5 Disorders of General Intelligence and Personality

General Intelligence

It is a general observation that intellectual activity falls off if the brain is severely damaged. This being so, it is often argued that the degree of intellectual fall-off seen in a person will reflect the extent of organic impairment. Is this so? In the previous chapters it has been noted that disruption of specific cerebral areas often causes the disruption of specific mental skills. A point that has perhaps not been mentioned very much hitherto, is that the loss of these skills does not inevitably reduce an individual's competence. The dysphasic patient can still communicate, the amnesic one uses a notebook or some other form of mnemonic to organize his daily life. Even the patient with visuo-perceptual disorders can compensate for his loss by developing new cues to orientate himself by. 'One can always use geometry,' said a world-famous mathematician, as he put the pieces of the WAIS Object Assembly together soon after having lost most of his right cerebral hemisphere as a result of a traffic accident.

Dementia and the effects of age

The tendency to compensate for changing mental skills is seen most clearly in the process of ageing (Welford, 1958). As people grow older, certain skills deteriorate. But the ageing person does not necessarily become a social burden. He may have difficulty remembering new names and faces due to his increasing age but this does not render him incapable of leading a useful social existence. He may have rigid 'old-fashioned' attitudes towards pop music and politics but be quite capable of running a household or even a business. He may be slow in his responses to changing signals but remain a safe car driver. A tendency to confuse the processes of normal ageing and of dementia have led to much muddled thinking. Hence a short summary of the similarities and differences between them may not be amiss. (For a fuller account see Williams, 1969.)

The effect of age is mostly seen in the spheres of speed (e.g. reaction time) and memory. The ability to deal with words

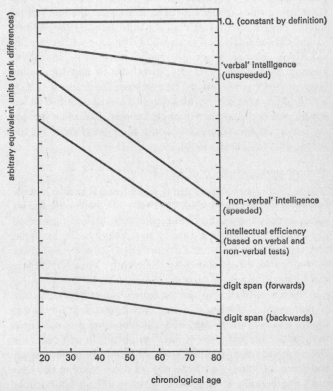

Figure 14 Age differences in the Wechsler–Bellevue functions expressed in equivalent units

falls off slowly, but the ability to manipulate visuo-construc-
tive tasks falls off comparatively soon. For this reason bat-
teries of tests (such as the WAIS, the Babcock, the Shipley–
Hertford, the Hunt–Minnesota) involving a variety of skills
show a characteristic pattern of subtest scatter with increasing
age, in which the untimed and information-measuring tests
(e.g. vocabulary, information, comprehension) *hold* whereas
those based on speed (digit symbol), learning (sentence
repetition), and visual construction (block design) *do not hold*
(see Figure 14). The degree of discrepancy shown between
these two groups of tests is taken to indicate the intellectual
fall-off present in the patient, but unfortunately they afford
no indication of the subject's ability to cope with everyday
situations. Nor is there any satisfactory way of making
allowance on these tests for past practice and life habits
(Piercy, 1959). As is only to be expected, the degree to which
a skill of any sort deteriorates depends on the extent to which
it was practised, so that it often happens that older people
do better on the reputedly 'don't hold' tests than on the
'hold' ones (Williams, 1960).

Dementia and the effects of focal lesions

In true intellectual deterioration or dementia the main trouble
lies, therefore, in the subject's inability to compensate for his
losses – not in the nature of the losses seen. Indeed signs of all
the specific impairments already noted (dysphasia, amnesia,
apraxia, etc.) may be present in generalized dementia but affect
over-all performance somewhat differently. These differences
can be summarized in Table 5.

A further difficulty in the assessment of general dementia
is that mental efficiency is influenced by many functional
illnesses as well as by age, and differentiation between these
in the older age groups is especially difficult. In particular the
older age groups not infrequently see the onset of depression
and paranoid illness, and the task of distinguishing between
these and organic derangements is often difficult but of great
clinical importance. A summary of the differences is shown in

Table 6. These signs do not always show up unless the subject is in an environment that elicits them. Hence tests in this case consist of a variety of tasks which a subject is asked to perform and which allow for his behaviour to be studied in a variety of fairly standardized situations.

Table 5

A Comparison of the Effects of Specific Disorders in Patients with Focal Lesions and those with Generalized Dementia

Disorders of memory (eliciting tests and situations: Benton's Designs from Memory Test, Wechsler's Memory Scale, Williams' Memory Scale)

	Focal lesions	*Dementia*
Abilities lost	Retention (especially of recent events) and learning in all sensory modalities	Retention, learning and some established skills
Orientation	Poor for time and place	Ditto
Insight	Often quite good	Usually poor
Mood	Usually euphoric	Agitated, perplexed, confused
Response to cues	Usually good, tendency to confabulate if very severe	Confabulation and distraction

Disorders of speech (eliciting tests and situations: Rochford and Williams' Scale for Measurement of Dysphasia, Eisenson's Dysphasia Test)

	Focal lesions	*Dementia*
Abilities lost	Expression and naming worse than comprehension.	Comprehension as bad or worse than expression.

Table 5 – *contd*

	Focal lesions	*Dementia*
	Reading aloud worse than recognition of written words. Errors indicate correct recognition of objects	Recognition of written words worse than reading aloud. Errors indicate misrecognition of objects
Orientation	Good	Poor
Insight	Good	Usually poor
Mood	Distressed by failure to find right words	Appears perfectly satisfied by own performance
Response to cues	Assisted by any semantic or mechanical lead-in	Distracted by all cues
Perseveration	Some words repeated in identical form despite *S*'s awareness of their irrelevance, e.g. chair = 'chair', book = 'chair. No! – chair'	Portions of words or phrases often carried over from one sentence to another with elaboration or correction, e.g. chair = 'a sitting on machine', book = 'a sitting on reading machine'

Disorders of perception (eliciting tests and situations: Bender–Gestalt, Block Construction, Picture Naming, Picture–Word Matching, walking around ward!)

	Focal lesions	*Dementia*
Abilities lost	Inability to appreciate whole or relationship between its parts although individual parts recognized	Whole object misidentified. Parts regarded as adequate wholes
Orientation	Spatial orientation poor. Orientation for time and person usually retained	All poor

Table 5 – *contd*

	Focal lesions	*Dementia*
Insight	S often perplexed and worried; feels 'something is wrong', but may attribute his difficulties to 'madness' or 'poor memory'	Little insight, S usually satisfied with performance
Mood	Perplexed and distressed when disorder elicited	Undisturbed by errors, but agitated if lost in ward
Response to cues	May be helped by verbal directions, and can often learn to orientate himself using verbal cues	Distracted and confused by cues

Disorders of motor skills (eliciting situations: dressing, tying a bow, lighting cigarette or candle, placing pegs in board)

	Focal lesions	*Dementia*
Abilities lost	Complicated sequencing of acts (apraxia)	Goal towards which act is directed
Abilities retained	Simple and automatic acts	Individual finger skills usually good
Orientation	Good	Poor
Insight	Good	Poor
Mood	Agitated by failure	Agitated when really confused, e.g. if clothes are on back to front
Response to cues	Little improvement unless complexity of situation is reduced. Verbal directions do not assist	Improvement if continually reminded of goal

Table 6

A Summary of Differences between Functional Illnesses and Organic Derangements in Old Age

Activity	Organic	Functional
Emotional expression	Labile, dependent on immediate stimulus	Consistent with internal preoccupations; unchanging
Psychomotor behaviour	Reaction time brisk, actions repetitive and stereotyped, tend to be restless, non-goal-orientated	Reaction time slow, little spontaneous activity, goal-orientated
Verbalization	Vocabulary and sentence structure usually intact, but statements contradictory or meaningless	Form intact, but content refers principally to preoccupations
Orientation	Poor for time and often also for place; orientation for person best retained	Usually intact, but may depend on preoccupation
Perception	Misperception evident in response to visual and verbal stimuli	Responds to external stimuli appropriately, despite pseudo-hallucinations and delusions

Other positive signs of general mental impairment which are liable to render a person incapable of compensating for specific losses and so lead to generalized intellectual deterioration are:

1. *Perseveration.* The patient repeats a response appropriate to one stimulus in response to the next one even when it is not appropriate to that. Thus asked to touch his nose, he does so correctly. Asked then to touch his ear, he again touches his nose. Asked to hold up his hand, he extends his fingers and places them on his nose.

Although perseveration may occur in association with any single cerebral lesion, it is most commonly seen in cases where the lesion is widespread and produces a variety of symptoms. Thus in all aphasics, some degree of perseveration is usually seen (Allison and Hurwitz, 1967) and is not correlated with any specific language defect. It is far commoner, however, in those showing jargon aphasia than in those with standard aphasia (Rochford, 1969). Perseveration in patients with dementia often takes the form of a repetition of a word or an idea in a slightly altered context.

2. *Stereotypy*. Allied to perseveration is inability to alter concepts, i.e. *stereotypy*. Seen particularly in the sort of situation where the subject has to categorize objects in a variety of different ways, it is found that once the subject has achieved one form of categorization he cannot adopt any others.

The Weigl–Goldstein–Scheerer Test which is a useful method for eliciting this behaviour consists of twelve pieces in three different shapes (triangle, circle, square) and four colours (red, blue, green, yellow). The subject is asked to sort these pieces into groups so that all the objects in each group are alike according to some principle, but are different to those in the other groups. Once a subject has sorted the pieces according to one principle (e.g. shape) they are jumbled up and he is asked to sort them again according to another. The organic patient can typically sort them according to one category but be quite unable to change his frame of reference at the second attempt. Instead of re-sorting them, he typically places them in patterns, all the triangles in one row, the squares below and the circles below that. Even if the examiner starts a group for him, he is likely to demolish it and revert to his previous system (Goldstein and Scheerer, 1941).

3. *Concreteness*. Another defect frequently shown up on sorting tests is that of *concreteness* – a tendency first described and named by Goldstein which may be evident in both verbal

and non-verbal performance. Concreteness is 'an attitude which is determined by, and cannot proceed beyond, some immediate experience, object or stimulus' (Mayer Gross, Slater and Roth, 1960). Thus a subject responds to all stimuli as if they existed only in the setting in which they are presented. He cannot abstract them from their environment or their qualities from them. A knife cannot be grouped with any other objects because it is different from them. A word cannot be defined properly as it fails to call up any other words. (Definitions, therefore, tend to consist of either repetitions or of sentences in which the word itself features, e.g. bed = 'Yes it's a bed. Well, just a bed you sleep on.' Breakfast = 'When you have your breakfast, you eat your breakfast – sometimes we have bacon and eggs.') Proverbs cannot be interpreted in terms of generalities but only in terms of the words they contain. (An interpretation of the proverb: 'Still waters run deep' was 'That's right; very deep and very still'.)

4. *Perplexity* is another sign of general intellectual impairment of organic origin first described by Goldstein (1939). Faced with a situation he cannot deal with, the patient tries to escape from it by indulging in irrelevant acts. Shown a picture he cannot name, he turns it over and looks on the back. Offered an object he cannot recognize, he puts it in his pocket or in his mouth.

5. *The catastrophic reaction* consists of an intense affective response with autonomic components (sweating, flushing, crying, restlessness) and has already been referred to. It is another typical response to a situation which cannot be coped with.

A number of suitable tests for eliciting these signs have been described by Goldstein and Scheerer in 1941 and consist of:

The cube test – the subject has to copy a number of designs in coloured cubes. The test is similar to the Kohs Blocks and to the block-design subtest of the Wechsler Scales.

Colour sorting test – woollen skeins of different hues and shades are presented to the subject who is asked to carry out a number of matching tasks with them.

The object-sorting test – the subject is presented with a large variety of common and toy objects and is asked to select an object and then pick out all the others which go with it, or group all the articles together in various ways.

The colour-sorting test (the Weigl–Goldstein–Scheerer Test). This has already been described above.

The Goldstein–Scheerer stick test – the subject is presented with a number of sticks of different length and is asked to copy designs made by the examiner, either beside the model or from memory.

The characteristic performance of patients with cerebral lesions have been described in detail by Goldstein and Scheerer and in more general outline by Williams (1965).

Psychological mechanisms

From the brief summary above it will be seen that the mental disorders leading to the patient's inability to compensate for his defect (i.e. the disorder which, therefore, underlies the condition referred to as general intellectual deterioration or dementia), are distinct from the skills dealt with in the previous sections. Although they are most often accompanied by some loss of skills, the defects described here may occur almost in isolation. They may even be recognized in a mild form which does not lead to complete loss of practical efficiency and may pass unrecognized unless the subject is put into the situations likely to elicit them. For example, a middle-aged woman was, until one week before her admission to hospital, a reliable and well-respected department manager in a large store. She had always been considered by her family to be an 'odd person' and when, some weeks before her admission, she began complaining of blackouts, dizzy spells, headaches and occasional lapses of memory, her relatives and colleagues took little note of her symptoms. It was only a careful neurological examination which revealed the nature of her illness, but even this showed little more than early signs of raised intracranial pressure. During a detailed psychological examination carried out in hospital before her operation, this patient completed all the subtests on the WAIS at the level expected of a person of her age and average I.Q. On a test of delayed recall (Williams, 1968) she showed some impairment, but it was not until she was asked to perform sorting tests that any definite disorder was noted. The patient sorted the Weigl quickly into shapes, but was quite incapable of switching from this categorization to colours. Even when the two red pieces were placed together and she was asked to complete this particular grouping, the patient was unable to do more than place all the other squares beside the red square and all the other circles beside the red circle.

The difficulty found by this patient, as by most of those with similar conditions, was not so much in forming an original classification as in letting go of it once it had been formed.

The psychological deficits described here seem to consist essentially of the breakdown of the mechanism whereby a person rejects the response first aroused by a stimulus (that most ready to hand) and replaces it by others more appropriate to the total situation. It is as if there is a failure of some filter through which reactions must pass before being put into operation.

Physiological mechanisms

Defects of the type mentioned in this chapter, if they are very gross, are always associated with widespread cerebral lesions. In their mildest form, they are traditionally ascribed to lesions of the frontal lobe, and in the case just described above a large frontal tumour was indeed found. But if this association with frontal lobe lesions is in fact the rule, the above defects should also follow the operation of pre-frontal leucotomy (see Figure 15) which is frequently carried out for the relief of psychotic or neurotic states.

The fact that they do so has been demonstrated in the two most systematic studies in this field. Partridge (1950) studied

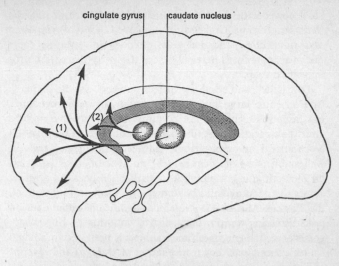

Figure 15 The fibre tracts interrupted in orbital leucotomy (1) and cingulectomy (2)

300 patients over a two-year period, and although he did not apply any standard psychological assessment procedures, the care he took in analysing and examining his data compensates for this lack. Considering only those patients who were regarded as having made a complete recovery from the mental illness precipitating the operation and only those in whom adequate pre-operative as well as post-operative information was available, Partridge was left with a small group of thirty-five patients on whom to draw conclusions regarding the effect of pre-frontal leucotomy on intellectual functions. Concreteness, a tendency to perseverate (e.g. to incorporate the set aroused by one stimulus into the response to the next), and reduced planning performance were seen in nearly all patients immediately post-operatively, together with 'less ready orientation in time', diminished power of rapidly altering the attention and some difficulty in holding several items in mind at the same time. These defects tended to be-

come fewer with the passage of time, but Partridge remarks that the patient's conversation remained 'factual, restricted and unreflective' and that gross difficulty in repeating digits backwards persisted in twenty-six of the thirty-five patients for up to two years.

Tow (1955) subjected a group of subjects, selected equally carefully, to a large battery of more standardized procedures, but his assessment did not continue beyond twelve months after the operation. He found significant falls on both verbal (vocabulary) and non-verbal (matrices) intelligence tests as well as on tasks of 'fluency' (the number of ideas triggered off by a stimulus), the ability to distinguish between abstract words (e.g. courage and boldness), an object-sorting test and the Porteus Mazes. He found no significant differences on tasks assessing tempo (the speed of counting and dressing), persistence (the length of time a subject is prepared to hold up his leg), speed-accuracy (cancellation or tracing) and reversal of letters.

Both these authors were struck more by the qualitative than by the quantitative changes in their subjects' behaviour. Thus on the vocabulary test the patient did not appear post-operatively to have forgotten words but Tow (1955) remarked, 'his short and often interrupted attempts never actually reached the point of definition. Usually the subject uses short phrases though he often repeats them.' In giving the difference between abstract words, the same tendency was seen. Examples quoted by Tow are given below:

Courage – you try to do a thing. Boldness – you can't do it. Thrift – you want more money. Avarice – you spend money. Murder – you kill a person. Manslaughter – you couldn't kill him.

It was, however, on the object-sorting test that Tow noted the most striking differences. The subject was presented with a tray full of common objects which could have been sorted according to four different principles – use, colour, material and shape. The first method of sorting, adopted by thirty-one people, was according to use. Twenty-one managed to sort according to colour, seventeen by material and twelve by shape. After the operation the number of people in each group fell significantly, but as well as this there was a striking tendency for most subjects to repeat their first sorting procedure over and over again, even though they might call it by a different name the second time and appear to believe that they had thereby found a new principle. Thus after putting the pen, pencil and ink together 'for writing' one subject when asked to sort them differently put the pen, pencil and protractor together 'for drawing'. Tow concludes (1955, p. 228):

There seems to be impairment in the powers of abstraction and synthesis; of perception of relations and differences; of the ability to deal with complex situations, planning, and thinking out the next action and its consequences; and appreciation of one's own mistakes. These are, of course, not several discrete functions but they are several closely related aspects of intellectual activity, which the tests show to be impaired.

A similar stereotypy and a tendency to adopt simple repetitive instead of more complex adaptive behaviour, has been noted by Luria, Karpor and Yarhuss (1966) in non-psychiatric patients with frontal lobe lesions. If a normal person is asked to differentiate by touch between the letters 'E' and 'H', he begins by feeling them extensively all over, but soon learns to single out the essential features. The original seeking movements and the subsequent abbreviation are both absent in frontal lobe patients, who repeat over and over their original rather cursory investigation and glibly give the first response that occurs to them. Again if such patients are asked to carry out motor activity based on the recoding of information (e.g. 'When I lift my finger you will show me your fist, and when I lift my fist you will show me your finger'), they soon replace the required act by simple imitation of the examiner's movements. Asked to lift his right hand after a single knock and his left hand after a double one, the frontal lobe patient quickly reverts to a stereotyped sequence of movements (R–L–R–L) irrespective of the signals (Luria, Karpor and Yarhuss, 1966).

The frontal lobes have been referred to up until now as if they formed one homogenous structure, but this is not the case. Pribram (1968) points out that to consider them as such,

may be one of the reasons for the confusion over their function. While the medial portion derives projections from the anterior thalamic nucleii, the polar and lateral portions receive projections from the midline of the thalamus and are reciprocally connected with the insular, amygdaloid and temporal cortices. Thus the frontal lobe can be divided into the medial, dorsolateral and posterior orbital sections. (See Figure 16.)

lateral surface   medial surface

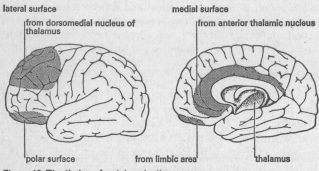

Figure 16 The thalamofrontal projection areas

In trying to associate psychological defects with the cerebral lesions producing them, Tow (1955, p. 236) concludes from his series of patients undergoing pre-frontal leucotomy:

The post-central area ... represents the more discriminative and more highly developed aspects of sensory function: the sensory cortex subserves all forms of discriminative sensation and the mechanisms by which all incoming sensory experiences are related to previous sensation. Similarly it seems that the pre-frontal area subserves not a few specific abilities, but rather the more discriminative and more highly developed aspects of them all.

No exact physiological mechanisms by which this last process is carried out was suggested by Tow nor by Partridge, but some hypotheses as to how they may be mediated are suggested at the end of this chapter.

In the above studies and in one conducted by Smith (1960), no difference between the function of the two frontal lobes was mentioned, but a later study reported by Smith (1966a) suggests that the two frontal lobes do reflect to some extent the specialization of the two hemispheres as a whole. Thus the left frontal lobe appears to be more concerned with linguistic than with visuo-spatial data, and the right vice versa. Benton (1968) confirms this finding and mentions that the defects shown by frontal lobe patients often reflect those shown by patients having post-rollandic lesions of the same hemisphere. In support of this hypothesis, Sylvester (1966) found a specific smallness of the parietal lobes, especially that associated with the posterior part of the callosal body, in the autopsy of eighty-four brains from subnormal subjects.

Experimental work with animals has not thrown as much light on the functions of the frontal lobes or on the factors underlying intellectual activity as might have been hoped, but it is nevertheless of some interest. Pribram has shown that lesions in the dorsolateral region in monkeys can be distinguished from those in other areas in respect to their effects on some aspects of learning and problem-solving behaviour.

Ever since experimental cerebral ablations of the frontal lobes have been carried out on monkeys, it has been noted that interference with the frontal lobe has impaired the animal's ability to perform the classical delayed retention problem – a task in which the animal has to remember, for specified periods, under which of two cups a reward has been placed. A 'normal' unoperated animal has no difficulty in retaining such information for long periods and will make few mistakes. The frontal lobe monkey, on the other hand, appears able to retain the information for only brief intervals. The reason for this difficulty, it has been demonstrated, is largely due to distractibility, perseveration or lack of attention to the cues (Mishkin and Pribram 1955, 1956.) It has further been shown by Yoshii (see Pribram and Tubbs, 1967) that animals with frontal ablations fail to show the same EEG responses to cues that are seen in normals learning the task.

Alternation problems – those in which the animal has to take his reward first from the right, then from the left and so on – are specifically failed by animals with lesions in the fronto-limbic formation, but not by those with lesions in the sensory–motor projection areas. But this apparently simple task *can* be solved by the frontal lobe preparations if each alternating pair (right–left) is separated from the next by a larger time interval. Thus the task, instead of being a continuous one – R–L–R–L – becomes 'parsed' or discontinuous – R–L . . . R–L . . . (Pribram and Tubbs, 1967).

From these observations, Pribram and Tubbs argue that one important function of the fronto-limbic areas may be that of 'chunking' incoming sensory information in such a way that it can be utilized to form a mental set. When the fronto-limbic area is removed, the chunking process has to be supplied from outside.

Personality

Personality can probably be viewed from as many different angles as there are viewers. It can be classified into as many different classes as there are classifiers, but by and large all these different attitudes can be divided into two main groups: those that consider the external manifestations of the person, i.e. his behaviour; and those that consider his internal structure, what makes him tick. The former is measured by traits and attitudes, the latter in terms of needs and drives. Psychometric assessment of the former is usually made by means of rating scales and questionnaires, while the latter is made by projective tests. The repertory grid and semantic differential techniques might claim to reflect both attitudes and needs to some extent.

Since any change in personality can only be seen by the observer in terms of altered behaviour, it is only the first of these aspects of personality which will be considered in this section although to explain behaviour it is often necessary to postulate inner mechanisms as well. Moreover, assessment of personality on the basis of traits and attitudes alone is not always reliable. There is considerable evidence that although these alter to some extent in the normal course of ageing, the ageing person does not change so much as he becomes more and more a caricature of his former self.

The first recorded and best-known instance of personality change resulting from physical injury was that described by Brickner in 1935. A farm labourer fell from a height onto a crowbar which penetrated his skull and destroyed a large part of his frontal lobes. The patient survived and made an apparently full physical recovery. From having been a conscientious, reliable, sober worker, the patient revealed all the opposite characteristics after recovery from his injury. He was uninhibited, unreliable, euphoric, lacking in judgement, childish and lazy. Similar changes had been seen by Rylander (1939) following tumours in the frontal region.

Most of the evidence concerning the personality changes following cerebral lesions comes, however, from studying patients on whom operations were performed for the relief of psychotic symptoms. Partridge's analysis of sixty fully recovered patients from thirty different mental hospitals in Great Britain, already referred to (Partridge, 1950), sums up the results of the first few years' findings most clearly.

Partridge divided his data on personality into three areas of function which he termed activity, affect and restraint. A summary of his findings 6 months, 12 months and 2 years post-operatively is shown in Table 7. The tendencies noted in these patients were not seen under all conditions. For example, if the social situation truly demanded it, a patient with marked loss of restraint could control himself and behave in a conventional manner. Partridge's findings have been criticized on two grounds: firstly, the operative technique to which these patients were subjected was a crude hit-and-miss affair, as a result of which the actual nature and extent of the lesions induced was often unknown. Secondly, the patients them-

Table 7

Personality Changes following Pre-Frontal Leucotomy (after Partridge, 1950)

Number of patients showing changes at varying post-operative times

	6 months	12 months	24 months
Activity			
More relaxed	52	41	?
Less active	49	33	?
Slower	44	37	15
Less spontaneous	41	18	12
Less persistent	39	34	28
Get up later	33	22	22
Combination of all above symptoms to some extent	60	56	52
Affect			
Worry less	60	54	?
Loss of 'feeling' for others	13	13 (less severe)	0
Fatuousness	12	7	?
Affect outwardly (but not subjectively) diminished	5	4	?
Less affectionate and more selfish	9	?	?
Restraint (Causing little concern to patient but much to relatives)	33	30	30
Snappishness	32	33	30
Selfishness	31	30	30
Bad temper	16	12	
Extravagance	15	15	15
Greedy	15	9	0
Bad language (swearing)	11	9	7
Inconsequential in conversation	11	14	?
Excessive smoking	7	4	4
Excessive alcohol intake	3	3	1
Violence	4	—	—

selves were suffering pre-operatively from a wide variety of mental and personality disorders, which had to be taken into account when the post-operative picture was considered. Lewin's (1961) observations overcome both these objections. He studied the effects of carefully controlled and circumscribed operations on patients with different and clearly defined pre-operative symptomatology. In one series of operations, he restricted his surgical procedure to undercutting the orbital surface of the frontal lobes thus only dividing the orbital cortex from the 'visceral brain' (orbital undercutting or orbital leucotomy). In another series, the anterior 4 centimetres of the cingulate gyrus was removed by suction on both sides, leaving the blood supply and the remainder of the frontal lobes intact (cingulectomy). (Figure 15, p. 135.)

Lewin considered his results only in relation to the pathological symptoms removed, not in relation to any other aspects of personality. It was clear from his paper, however, that while symptoms of severe psychotic disorders (including schizophrenic illness) were not influenced basically by either procedure, orbital undercutting was very effective in removing symptoms of anxiety and depression, while cingulectomy was effective in removing aggression and obsessional disorders. In the latter operation, it was not so much the habit which was disrupted as the emotional state associated with it. This was illustrated by one patient seen by the present author who had developed a ritual in which he had to hold onto every movable object he touched (and who thus collected onto his person an immense and ever-growing mountain of rubbish such as empty bottles, cutlery and cigarette ends). After the operation the patient remarked: 'I still sometimes find myself collecting things but now I just say to myself, "Well, you had the operation, you can throw them away and you won't worry", and I do and I'm all right.'

Petrie (1958) has compared the effects of a variety of different operative and pharmacological procedures on patients with different pre-operative symptoms and personality profiles, including patients treated for intractable pain rather than mental disorder. The findings are not always easy to follow, as she divides all her subjects along the dimensions of introversion and neuroticism (after Eysenck, 1947) and considers her results in relation only to these dimensions. She concludes that after pre-frontal leucotomy the subject becomes more extroverted. Hence leucotomy is likely to be (as is found to be the case) most effective in those subjects who were pre-operatively introverted. Local operations on specific areas of the frontal lobes (including orbital undercutting) were found to produce the same changes as leucotomy but to a lesser extent. Cingulectomy, on the other hand, was found to increase the scores suggesting introversion and was only effective in subjects who were originally low on these scores. Petrie claims that temporal lobectomy carried out for the relief of epilepsy, as well as administration of chlorpromazine, has the same effect as cingulectomy. She also claims that the effects of stereotactic operations causing coagulation of the anterior nucleus of the thalamus are different from those causing coagulation of the dorsomedial nucleus, the former resembling the effect of cingulectomy while the latter resemble those of pre-frontal leucotomy.

In subjects suffering from intractable pain, Petrie (1960a and b) found that leucotomy only gave relief to patients who originally showed high introversion scores, the relief being relative to the extent that the patients were rendered more extroverted. Petrie's explanation for these various findings and the mechanisms postulated by her will be considered later, but it may be mentioned in passing that her finding that orbital leucotomy increases extroversion has not been substantiated by Levinson and Meyer (1965). The latter authors claim that increases are only seen in those people whose pre-operative scores were low and thus the observations show little more than a 'regression towards the mean' – a characteristic of any test repetition.

Another psychosurgical procedure whose results are of considerable interest is selective electrocoagulation described by Crow, Cooper and Phillips (1963) as follows:

Electrode sheaves are inserted through two frontal burr holes so as to lie in fans in both frontal lobes. . . . The aim is to produce controlled multifocal frontal leucotomy. After subsidence of the insertion effects, records are obtained for several days from all electrodes to eliminate the possibility of local pathology. The functional positions of the electrodes in relation to grey and white matter are then established by graded stimulation. Electrodes lying in cortical convolutions exhibit characteristic after-discharges at a threshold of about 4 volts, while those in white matter show no after-discharges at twice or thrice this level. From this information a chart of the electrodes in relation to cortical grey matter is prepared; attention is restricted to those in white matter.

The preliminary treatment is by polarization. The effects of polarization are brief but sometimes dramatic in relief of specific symptoms. The preliminary trials may last several weeks, since fifty or so electrodes may lie in frontal white matter and several days may be necessary to follow the temporary change in condition. When electrodes giving favourable results with polarization have been identified, the current is raised to a level known to produce electrolytic coagulation and this is applied to each electrode in turn, again with periods of several days intervening to determine the extent of clinical remission.

Psychological mechanisms

In considering the clinical changes actually brought about by psychosurgical procedures, a great deal of confusion may result from the fact that the concepts underlying the use of certain terms differ among different people. Walter (1966) stresses the fact that selective coagulation procedures have only been employed on patients who were carefully selected for 'good previous personality'. Indeed the importance of previous personality in determining the effect of psychosurgical procedures has been stressed by nearly all workers. But what is a 'good personality'? Birley (1964), trying to define the term, found it extremely difficult. The only feature consistent amongst all his 106 cases was an absence of 'bad personality' features, among which he included aggression, bad work record, and addiction (see also Marks, Birley and Gelder 1966).

Green *et al.* (1958), trying to analyse the personality changes following temporal lobectomy (for the relief of epilepsy), managed to clarify their findings by summarizing the changes noted under the three headings of thinking, feeling and acting. In 80 per cent of the cases they noted considerable improvement in feeling or affect; acting improved in conjunction with it, although alterations to thinking were negligible. They suggest that much of the improvement they did find may have been due to 'stabilization because of increased security in the environment', rather than any actual alteration to cerebral function. However, even when such global terms as 'personality' are replaced by more specific ones, difficulties may still arise. Even the concentration on symptoms may not solve all the problems. Much stress has been laid by clinicians on the fact that frontal lesions affect specifically aggressiveness, spontaneity and anxiety but, as Costello (1966) points out, what the clinician understands by these words may be very different from that understood by experimentalists. Costello himself (in line with the majority of psychologists) prefers to consider behaviour under two headings: the actions observed and the conditions associated with them. For example, if the satisfaction of a primary drive is frustrated, the individual may react by blaming himself, blaming someone else, stereotyped repetitive activity, regression to a more primitive mode of behaviour or physiological (autonomic) signs of stress. Again, if an individual is faced with an unharmonious, inconsistent, discrepant relationship between two events (the cognitive dissonance of Festinger, 1957, or the double-bind situation of Bateson *et al.*, 1956), he may minimize or ignore one of them, increase or add to the other, or opt out of the situation by minimizing the importance of both.

It is, of course, apparent that different people tend to do different things in the same situation, and that the same people may do different things in different situations. However, since behaviour of this type is objectively measurable, at least all observers do know that they are dealing with the same phenomena when discussing them.

Unfortunately the effects of psychosurgical procedures and of frontal lesions have never been studied in relation to carefully controlled situations such as frustration tolerance or cognitive dissonance: such studies might well be worth carrying out and might reveal interesting new data.

Physiological mechanisms

It has been fairly traditional to explain the connexion between the frontal lobes and personality structure on the basis of 'long circuiting' of sensory impressions – a hypothesis first put forward by Cobb (1952). Greenblatt and Solomon (1958) quote in support of this suggestion the almost invariable sequences to frontal lobe damage of (a) a reduction in drive or energy, (b) the subject is less affected by past experience and more bound to immediate stimuli and (c) he is less able to elaborate experience or sustain experiences. 'One way of looking at this,' they conclude, 'is that the mechanism of prolongation in time is impaired.'

Closer investigation over the past years has, however, led to some modification of this view. In the first place the realization that identical procedures may lead to different results in different types of people has led to the conclusion that some different form of explanation is required. For example, Petrie (1960a) found that leucotomy for the relief of pain had different results not only in relation to the subject's pre-operative dimension of introversion but also in relation to the subject's responses to perceptual satiation. Thus if subjects are presented with a sensory stimulus for a certain time (e.g. asked to handle an object of a specific thickness) and then asked to make a judgement of its intensity (e.g. match the test object with others of the same subjective thickness), it is found that people generally can be divided into the augmentors and the reducers. The augmentors are those who tend to match the block with one thicker than itself, the reducers to one thinner. Augmentors also tend to be what Petrie calls extroverts, reducers to be introverts.

Tolerance to pain is generally greater in the reducers than

in the augmentors. This is explained on the basis that 'a brief wave of intense pain could cause later pain to appear less severe' (Petrie, 1960a). It will be remembered that relief from pain was only produced in those subjects who also showed increased extroversion after the operation. Since neither increased extroversion nor relief from pain are brought about by cingulectomy, temporal lobectomy or orbital undercutting, Petrie argues that a 'centre' for the processing and assimilating of incoming sensory data is probably present in the prefrontal lobes, which above all areas of the brain are specialized to carry out this function.

Walter (1966) comes to a somewhat similar conclusion from completely different data. Studying the EEG records from the scalp over the frontal lobes which follow when two signals occur together over a number of trials, Walter found that a characteristic response (the contingent negative variation, CNV, or expectancy wave) occurred between the two signals. He continues:

Our most exciting discovery is that when a person has to take some action, physical or mental (if there is a distinction), in response to the second or later signal, a dramatic change appears in the electrical state of the frontal cortex. As the association of signals is repeated and the action performed, a new effect appears: a slow rise in the negative potential of the cortex that starts just after the first signal and continues until the moment of action or decision when it terminates abruptly.

We have found the CNV or E-wave in a wide variety of situations. The simplest is in the establishment of a 'classical' blink, conditioned reflex when a click is followed by a puff of air to the eye. In this case the E-wave tends to appear during acquisition but declines when the conditional response is well established (Walter, 1967, p. 259).

Studying the CNV in many patients before and after prefrontal leucotomy, Walter (1966) found that habituation of the CNV did not occur in patients with chronic anxiety or phobic states: the CNV is almost absent in psychopaths and those who seem unable to learn from society, while in the obsessional patient it not only fails to habituate if the second signal is not reinforced, but may even increase its original amplitude. In psychotic subjects, especially schizophrenics, the results are irregular. Electrocoagulative leucotomy, where it successfully relieves symptoms, is usually followed by return of the CNV to the normally adaptive pattern.

When considering what the CNV represents, Walter (1967) points out that it is essentially related to uncertainty.

In many people there is an almost linear relation between the maximum potential reached by the E-wave and the arithmetical probability of signal association. This means that in such people the subjective probability and objective probability coincide. A very interesting complication appears here however. The E-wave does not of course appear at once when an association of signals for action is presented; it grows steadily over a certain number of experiences. This number is usually (again in normal adult subjects) about twenty-five when the presentations are irregular at about one every 5 to 10 seconds. This means that the brain must, quite reasonably, acquire a certain number of samples before it 'decides' that subjective certainty is attained. In ordinary life, if two events occur together twenty-five times running, one would probably consider their association a pretty trustworthy basis for action. However, the criterion of certainty as indicated by number of trials to E-wave plateau is a very personal factor. This means that, in effect, the brain computes a running average of associations, and if one takes the number of trials needed for full development of the E-wave as the personal criterion of certainty used by a particular brain the effects of uncertainty and of stress come out very tidily.

Thus, for Walter, the frontal lobes of the brain act not just as long circuiters but as highly skilled computers, calculating probabilities and preparing the rest of the body to take appropriate action. He maintains indeed that variations in evoked response patterns and CNV lead to the tentative identification of three main systems subserved by the frontal lobes.

One is related to the limbic regions and serves primarily as a warning system – 'Something has happened.' Excessive or persistent activity in this system leads to the feeling, 'everything is happening at once'. Another system seems to involve more directly the cingulate structures and is concerned with the maintenance of conditional attention. 'This may be worth remembering.' Here, overactivity results in persistent recall and cyclic compulsion – 'I can't get it out of my head.' The third system, engaging mainly superior frontal neocortex, provides the conceptual linkage between events – 'There must be some connexion between these experiences.' Exaggeration or persistence of this process leads to superstitious conviction – 'I don't care what you say, *I know.*' [See Figure 17.]

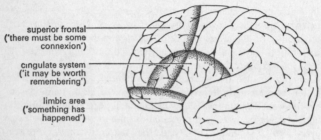

superior frontal
('there must be some
connexion')

cingulate system
('it may be worth
remembering')

limbic area
('something has
happened')

Figure 17 Functional areas of frontal lobes

Such a conclusion is very attractive. It satisfies man's innate desire to avoid uncertainty. Even if we have to accept that all sensory knowledge merely results from calculations based on probabilities, at least to know whereabouts in our bodies these calculations are carried out is comforting. But even if correct, this conclusion still does not solve all the problems of personality and its physiological basis. To take but one example of the confusing findings which still have to be explained, one of the first physiological results of stress and anxiety is autonomic arousal, and recently it has been found that a reliable measure of this is the amount of blood flowing down the forearm. Kelly, Walter and Sargeant (1966) studied the forearm bloodflow in a number of patients treated by modified leucotomy. After the operation all measures of anxiety fell as did also the forearm bloodflow. However, it was found that clinical improvement was not necessarily related to either of these measures, and in particular high preoperative forearm bloodflow was not in itself a particularly good indicator of clinical recovery.

Conclusions

From the examples of behaviour described in the preceding pages it will be clear that organic cerebral dysfunction does not cause all psychological activity to stop. Far from ceasing, activity is sometimes even over-abundant; it is its relevance to external stimuli which is most commonly at fault.

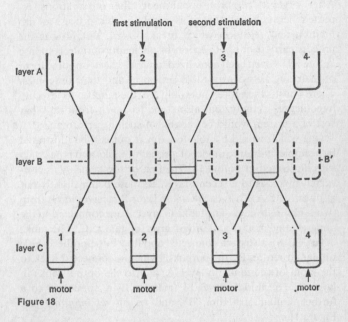

Figure 18

The most frequent observation is that reactions are made which, although acquired from past experience, are inappropriate in the given circumstances and would probably be inhibited or modified by the healthy individual. They are near approximations to those actually required, the pool from which the desired would be drawn.

It is cogently argued in the theory of microgenesis (Werner, 1956) that all normal or healthy stimulus–response behaviour begins with the arousal of a general pool of relatively appropriate behaviour (the *Vor Gestalt*), and that before the most appropriate response can be made, this pool has to be carefully sifted. The inappropriate responses have to be rejected (their threshold to production thereby being raised) before the most appropriate can be selected. It is via the rejection of the inappropriate responses that the appropriate one is selected. After organic cerebral impairment, the observations reported here suggest that it is precisely this process of inhibition and rejection which breaks down. But how is the process carried out? Rejection of an inappropriate response before it has even been actualized, must be based on some form of matching between possible responses and their outcomes. There must, therefore, not only be the ability to execute hypothetical activity, but also some feedback from it. What sort of a system would be capable of such a performance?

One which would be able to carry it out can be illustrated by a simple hydraulic model of a series of tanks and pipes such as is illustrated in Figure 18. The first or top layer, A, is connected by pipes to a second layer, B, these being slightly out of phase with A. Thus each tank in layer B receives input from two tanks in layer A. The tanks in layer B are connected in the same arrangement to a further layer of tanks, C. The tanks in layer B are also each connected and flow into another whole similar structure, B', the output of which is connected back to the input of the tanks in layer A, and to the output tanks in layer C. The middle layer of tanks in B' is connected to a further similar structure, B'', and so on *ad infinitum* (see Figure 19).

Now consider that some water is poured into tank 2 in layer A, Figure 18. The water will flow into the two tanks connected to tank A2 in layer B, and from those into the three tanks connected to them in layer C. The motors connected to these three tanks (C1, 2 and 3) will then be set in motion. Some water will also flow into the tanks in B'. The level of water in all these tanks will be raised and, if the pipes leaving these tanks do so at a point slightly above the ground level, some

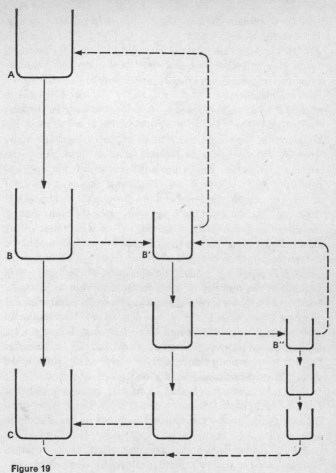

Figure 19

water will remain in these tanks after it has ceased to flow through the whole system.

Now consider that water is poured into tank A3, Figure 18. It will flow as before, but as a result of the previous 'stimulation' of the system via tank 2, power will be driven into the motors connected to tanks C2 and 3 before it reaches a critical level in tanks C1 and 4. It can be said that the stimulation of tank 2 has left a 'memory' which is reflected in the behaviour of the whole unit. The same process repeated many times over in systems B' and B" will leave an impression in the whole system which might cause the sort of integration, suppression and selection of behaviour seen in normal states. The degree of arousal and retention in the system would depend on the width of the pipes connecting the tanks and on the distance up the sides of the tanks from which these pipes leave. Both these factors may depend on, and would be influenced by, the elasticity of the material with which both tanks and pipes are made. The efficiency of the system will depend on the number of units functioning in it as a whole, and particularly on those further away from the main stimulus response area, A to C, i.e. it will depend on the complexity of systems B' and B". Should these be reduced in quantity, only those responses immediately evoked by a stimulus applied to a particular tank in layer A will result. Integration with past experience will be lacking.

Thus selection and rejection of possible behaviour patterns and the qualitative differences within behaviour is reduced to a quantitative basis – a situation which has its parallel in the sensory field. For example, it is well known that after injury to the peripheral nerves, the first stage of returning sensation consists of a general awareness (protopathic sensitivity) without the subject being able to differentiate heat, pain or touch. Only later do these more specific qualitative differences (epicritic sensation) return. Henry Head believed that two distinct systems had to be evoked to account for such great qualitative effects, but it has been established by later workers that the difference is purely quantitative – 'protopathic characteristics being due to the response of a relatively thinned out mosaic of receptor' (Fulton, 1949).

The system of tanks and pipes put forward here as a model for mental behaviour is crude in the extreme. Modern computers carry out a similar task in more refined ways, but the task is essentially the same. The major advantage of the computer model is that its activities can be defined mathematically.

These models, however, all suggest that mental activity can be reduced to one single process which is repeated over and over again in different units or bundles of units. How it is that when carried out by the frontal lobes they become thoughts, inhibitions, abstractions and foresight, when carried out by the parietal lobes they become visuomotor perceptions and when carried out by the temporal lobes they become memory and speech, we are still far from explaining. Replacing the jargon of phenomenology by that of differential calculus has not completely solved the problem, although it may have given us better tools with which to work on it. Neuropsychologists can take comfort, however, from the fact that not only the physiologists but even more material scientists are in something of the same dilemma. The seat of a chair and the point of a sword can both be reduced in a final physical analysis to empty space held together by electrical forces – but they are very different things to sit upon.

References

ABERCROMBIE, M. L. J. (1960), 'Perception and eye movements in cerebral palsy', *Cer. Palsy Bull.*, vol. 2, p. 142.

ALAJOUANINE, T., and L'HERMITTE, F. (1965), 'Acquired aphasia in children', *Brain*, vol. 88, p. 44.

ALLISON, R. S., and HURWITZ, L. J. (1967), 'On perseveration in aphasia', *Brain*, vol. 90, p. 429.

ARCHIBALD, Y. M., and WEPMAN, J. M. (1968), 'Language disturbances and non-verbal cognition', *Brain*, vol. 91, p. 117.

BATESON, G., JACKSON, D. D., HALEY, J., and WEAKLAND, J. (1956), 'Towards a theory of schizophrenia', *Behav. Sci.*, vol. 1, p. 251.

BENDER, M. B., and DIAMOND, S. P. (1965), 'Auditory perceptual defects and localization of function', *Brain*, vol. 88, p. 675.

BENTON, A. (1968), 'Differential behavioural effects of frontal lobe disease', *Neuropsychol.*, vol. 6, p. 53.

BIRCH, H. G., BELMONT, I., and KARP, E. (1967), 'Delayed processing and extinction', *Brain*, vol. 90, p. 113.

BIRLEY, J. L. T. (1964), 'Modified leucotomy – a review of 106 cases', *Brit. J. Psychiat.*, vol. 110, p. 211.

BLAKEMORE, C. B., and FALCONER, M. A. (1967), 'Long-term effects of anterior temporal lobectomy', *J. Neurol. Neurosurg. Psychiat.*, vol. 30, p. 364.

BOLLER, F., and VIGNOLO, L. A. (1966), 'Latent sensory aphasia', *Brain*, vol. 89, p. 815.

BRICKNER, R. M. (1935), *Intellectual Functions of the Frontal Lobes*, Macmillan, New York.

BRIERLEY, J. B. (1966), 'The neuropathology of amnesic states', in C. W. M. Whitty and O. L. Zangwill (eds.), *Amnesia*, Butterworth, ch. 7.

BROMLEY, D. B. (1966), *The Psychology of Human Ageing*, Penguin.

CAIRNS, H. (1952), 'Disturbances of consciousness in lesions of the mid-brain and diencephalon', *Brain*, vol. 75, p. 109.

CAIRNS, H., and TAYLOR, M. (1949), 'Tuberculous meningitis', *Proc. Roy. Soc. Med.*, vol. 42, p. 155.

CLARDY, E. R., and HILL, B. C. (1949), 'Sleep disorders in institutionalised children', *Nerv. Child.*, vol. 8, p. 50.

157 References

COBB, S. (1952), *Foundations of Neuropsychiatry*, Williams & Wilkins.

CONRAD, R. (1964), 'Acoustic confusion in immediate memory', *Brit. J. Psychol.*, vol. 55, p. 75.

CORDEAU, J. P., and MAHERT, H. (1964), 'Temporal lobe resection in monkeys', *Brain*, vol. 87, p. 117.

COSTELLO, C. G. (1966), *Psychology for Psychiatrists*, Pergamon.

CRITCHLEY, M. (1953), *The Parietal Lobes*, Edward Arnold.

CRITCHLEY, M. (1965), 'Acquired anomalies of colour', *Brain*, vol. 88, p. 71

CROW, H. J., COOPER, R., and PHILLIPS, D. G. (1963), *Progressive Leucotomy in Current Psychiatric Therapies*, Grune & Stratton.

CURRY, F. K. W. (1967), 'Handedness and dichotic listening tasks', *Cortex*, vol. 3, p. 343.

CURRY, F. K. W., and RUTHERFORD, D. R. (1967), 'Recognition and recall of dichotically presented verbal stimuli', *Neuropsychol.*, vol. 5, p. 119.

DE RENZI, E., FAGLIONI, P., and SPINNLER, H. (1968), 'Face recognition and brain damage', *Cortex*, vol. 4, p. 17.

DE RENZI, E., and VIGNOLO, L. A. (1962), 'A token test for the measurement of psyphasia', *Brain*, vol. 85, p. 665.

DE RENZI, E., PIECZURO, A., and VIGNOLO, L. A. (1968), 'Ideational apraxia; a quantitative study', *Neuropsychol.*, vol. 6, p. 41.

EFRON, R. (1963), 'Perception of simultaneity', *Brain*, vol. 86, pp. 261, 285.

ERVIN, F R. (1967), 'Epilepsy', in A. M. Freedman and H. I. Kaplan (eds.), *Comprehensive Textbook of Psychiatry*, Williams & Wilkins, ch. 21.

ETTLINGER, G. (1960), 'Interpretation of pictures in cases of brain lesion', *J. ment. Sci.*, vol. 106, p. 1337.

ETTLINGER, G., and WYKE, M. (1961), 'Defects in identification in cerebrovascular disease', *J. Neurol. Neurosurg. Psychiat.*, vol. 24, p. 254.

EYSENCK, H. J. (1947), *Dimensions of Personality*, Routledge & Kegan Paul.

FESTINGER, L. (1957), *A Theory of Cognitive Dissonance*, Stanford University Press.

FREIDMAN, A. M., and KAPLAN, H. I. (1967), *Comprehensive Textbook of Psychiatry*, Williams & Wilkins.

FREUD, S. (1891), *On Aphasia*, trans. E. Stengel, Imago, 1950.

FULTON, J. (1949), *Textbook of Physiology*, Saunders, 16th edn.

GAZZANIGA, M. S., and SPERRY, R. W. (1967), 'Language after section of the cerebral commissures', *Brain*, vol. 90, p. 131.

GAZZANIGA, M. S., BOGAN, J. E., and SPERRY, R. W. (1965), 'Disconnexion of the cerebral hemispheres', *Brain*, vol. 88, p. 221.

GERTSMANN, J. (1924), 'Finger agnosia', *Wien Klin. Wschr.*, vol. 37, p. 1010.

GESCHWIND, N. (1965), 'Disconnection syndromes in animals and men', *Brain*, vol. 88, p. 237.

GHENT-BRAINE, L. (1968), 'Asymmetries of pattern perception in Israelis', *Neuropsychol.*, vol. 6, p. 73.

GIBBS, F. A. (1958), 'Abnormal electrical activity in the temporal region and abnormalities of behavior', in *The Brain and Human Behavior*, Association for Research in Nervous and Mental Disease, Illinois, ch. 10 (Hafner edn 1966).

GLONING, T., GLONING, K., and HOFF, H. (1968), *Neuropsychological Symptoms and Occipital Lesions*, Gauthier-Villars.

GLONING, I., GLONING, K., HOFF, H., and TSCHABITSCHER, H. (1966), 'Zur Prosopagnosie', *Neuropsychol.*, vol. 4, p 113.

GLONING, K., HARB, G., and QUATEMBER, R. (1966), 'Untersuchung der Prosopagnosie', *Neuropsychol.*, vol. 5, p. 99.

GOLDSTEIN, K. (1939), *The Organism*, American Book Co.

GOLDSTEIN, K. (1948), *Language and Language Disturbances*, Grune & Stratton.

GOLDSTEIN, K., and SCHEERER, M. (1941), 'Abstract and concrete behavior', *Psychol. Monog.*, vol. 53, no. 2.

GOODGLASS, H., and KAPLAN, E. (1963), 'Disturbances of gesture and pantomime in aphasia', *Brain*, vol. 86, p. 703.

GORDON, N., and TAYLOR, J. G. (1966), 'Children with difficulties of communication', *Brain*, vol. 87, p. 121.

GREEN, J. R., STEDMAN, H. F., DUISBERG, R. E. H., McGRATH, W. B., and WICK, S. W. (1958), 'Behavior changes following temporal lobe excision', in *The Brain and Human Behavior*, Association for Research in Nervous and Mental Disease, Illinois, ch. 11 (Hafner edn 1966).

GREENBLATT, M., and SOLOMON, H. C. (1958), 'Studies in lobotomy', in *The Brain and Human Behavior*, Association for Research in Nervous and Mental Disease, Illinois, ch. 2 (Hafner edn 1966).

HALLIDAY, A. M., DAVISON, K., BROWNE, M. W., and KREEGER, L. C. (1968), 'A comparison of bilateral and unilateral ECT', *Brit. J. Psychiat.*, vol. 114, p. 997.

HALNAN, C. R. E., and WRIGHT, G. H. (1961), 'Fingers and toes in the body image', *Acta Neurol. Scand.*, vol. 37, p. 50.

HEAD, H. (1926), *Aphasia and Kindred Disorders of Speech*, vol. 1, Cambridge University Press.

HERBERG, J. (1967), 'The hypothalamus and the aetiology of the migraine syndrome', in R. Smith (ed.) *Background to Migraine*, Heinemann.

HOWES, D. H., and GESCHWIND, N. (1961), Statistical properties of aphasic language, *Excerpta Medica Int. Cong. Ser.*, no. 38 (VIIth International Congress of Neurology).

HUMPHREY, M. E., and ZANGWILL, O. L. (1952), 'Effects of right-sided occipitoparietal brain injury in a left-handed man', *Brain*, vol. 75, p. 312.

HUTT, C., and COXON, M. W. (1965), 'Systematic observation on clinical psychology', *Arch. gen. Psychiat.*, vol. 12, p. 374.

HUTT, C., HUTT, J. T., LEE, D., and OUNSTED, C. (1964), 'Arousal in childhood autism', *Nature*, vol. 204, p. 908.

JACKSON, J. H. (1866), 'Notes on the physiology and pathology of language', reprinted in J. Taylor (ed.), *Selected Papers*, vol. 2, Hodder & Stoughton, 1932.

JAMBOR, K., and WILLIAMS, M. (1964), 'Disorders of topographical orientation', *Neuropsychol.*, vol. 2, p. 55.

KELLY, D. H. W., WALTER, C. J. S., and SARGEANT, W. (1966), 'Modified leucotomy assessed by forearm bloodflow', *Brit. J. Psychiat.*, vol. 112, p. 871.

KIMURA, D. (1963), 'Visual perception by patients with temporal lobe lesions', *Arch. Neurol. Chicago*, vol. 8, p. 264.

KIMURA, D. (1964), 'Left–right differences in the perception of melodies', *Quart. J. exp. Psychol.*, vol. 16, p. 355.

KIMURA, D. (1967), 'Asymmetry of the brain in visual perception', *Neuropsychol.*, vol. 4, p. 275.

KING, E. (1967), 'The nature of visual field defects', *Brain*, vol. 90, p. 647.

KINSBOURNE, M., and WARRINGTON, E. K. (1962), 'Reading loss associated with hemisphere lesions', *J. Neurol. Neurosurg. Psychiat.*, vol. 25, p. 339.

KINSBOURNE, M., and WARRINGTON, E. K. (1963a), 'Limited visual form perception', *Brain*, vol. 86, p. 697.

KINSBOURNE, M., and WARRINGTON, E. K. (1963b), 'A study of visual perseveration', *J. Neurol. Neurosurg. Psychiat.*, vol. 26, p. 468.

KINSBOURNE, M., and WARRINGTON, E. K. (1963c), 'Jargon aphasia', *Neuropsychol.* vol. 1, p. 27.

KINSBOURNE, M., and WARRINGTON, E. K. (1964), 'Disorders of spelling', *J. Neurol. Neurosurg. Psychiat.*, vol. 27, p. 224.

LANCASTER, N. P., STEINERT, R. R., and FROST, I. (1958), 'Unilateral ECT', *J. ment. Sci.*, vol. 104, p. 221.

LASHLEY, K. S. (1950), 'In search of the engram', *Symp. exp. Biol.*, vol. 4, p. 454.

LEVINSON, F., and MEYER, V. (1965), 'Personality changes following orbital cortex undercutting', *Brit. J. Psychiat.*, vol. 111, p. 207.

LEWIN, W. W. (1961), 'Observations on selective leucotomy', *J. Neurol. Neurosurg. Psychiat.*, vol. 24, p. 37.

LEWIN, W. W. (1968), 'Rehabilitation of head injuries', *Brit. med. J.*, vol. 1, p. 465.

LURIA, A. R. (1966), *Human Brain and Psychological Processes*, Harper & Row.

LURIA, A. R., KARPOR, B. A., and YARHUSS, A. L. (1966), 'Disturbances of visual perception in frontal lesions', *Cortex*, vol. 2, p. 202.

MARKS, I. M., BIRLEY, J. L. T., and GELDER, M. G. (1966), 'Modified leucotomy in severe agoraphobia', *Brit. J. Psychiat.*, vol. 112, p. 757.

MAYER GROSS, W. (1943), 'Memory defects after ECT', *Lancet*, vol. 2, p. 603.

MAYER GROSS, W., SLATER, E., and ROTH, M. (1960), *Clinical Psychology*, Cassell.

MCFIE, J., PIERCY, M. F., and ZANGWILL, O. L. (1950), 'Visuo-spatial agnosia', *Brain*, vol. 73, p. 167.

MCGHIE, A., CHAPMAN, J., and LAWSON, J. S. (1965), 'The effect of distraction on schizophrenic performance', *Brit. J. Psychiat.*, vol. 3, pp. 383, 391.

MCKINNEY, J. P. (1967), 'Handedness, eyedness and perceptual stability', *Neuropsychol.*, vol. 5, p. 339.

MILES, T. R. (1967), 'In defence of the concept of dyslexia', in J. Downing and A. L. Brown (eds.), *The Second International Reading Symposium*, Cassell.

MILNER, B. (1962), 'Laterality effects in audition', in V. B. Mountcastle (ed.), *Interhemispheric Relations and Cerebral Dominance*, Johns Hopkins University Press.

MILNER, B. (1966), 'Amnesia following operations on the temporal lobe', in C. W. M. Whitty and O. L. Zangwill (eds.), *Amnesia*, Butterworth, ch. 5.

MISHKIN, M., and PRIBRAM, K. H. (1955, 1956), 'The effects of frontal lesions in monkeys. I', *J. comp. physiol. Psychol.*, vol. 48, p. 492; 'II', ibid., vol. 49, p. 36.

MITCHELL, S. W. (1871), 'Phantom limbs', *Lippincotts Mag. pop. lit. Sci.*, vol. 8, p. 563.

NEWCOMBE, F., and MARSHALL, J. C. (1966), 'Syntatic and semantic errors in paralexia', *J. Neurol. Psychol.*, vol. 4, p. 169.

NEWCOMBE, F. and MARSHALL, J. C. (1967), 'Immediate recall of sentences by subjects with unilateral lesions', *Neuropsychol.*, vol. 5, p. 329.

OJEMANN, G. A., FEDIO, P., and VAN BUREN, J. M. (1968),

'Anomia from pulvinar and subcortical parietal stimulation', *Brain*, vol. 91, p. 29.

OLDFIELD, R. C., and WINGFIELD, A. (1965), 'Response latencies in naming objects', *Quart. J. exp. Psychol.*, vol. 16, p. 273.

OLDS, J. (1958), 'Self-stimulation experiments and reward systems', reprinted in D. Bindra and J. Stewart (eds.), *Motivation*, Penguin, 1966.

ORBACH, J. (1967), 'Recognition of English and Hebrew words in the right and left visual fields', *Neuropsychol.*, vol. 5, p. 127.

OSWALD, I. (1966), *Sleep*, Penguin.

OTTOSON, J. O. (1960), 'The action of ECT', *Acta Psychiat. Scand.*, supp. 145.

PARTRIDGE, M. (1950), *Prefrontal Leucotomy*, Blackwell.

PENFIELD, W., and BOLDREY, E. (1937), 'Somatic and sensory representation in the cortex of man', *Brain*, vol. 60, p. 432.

PENFIELD, W., and PEROT, P. (1963), 'The brain's record of auditory and visual experience', *Brain*, vol. 86, p. 595.

PETRIE, A. (1958), 'The effects of chlorpromazine and brain lesions on personality', in H. D. Pennes (ed.), *Psychopharmacology*, Hoeber-Harper.

PETRIE, A. (1960a), 'Some psychological aspects of pain', *Ann. N.Y. Acad. of Sc.*, vol. 86, p. 13.

PETRIE, A. (1960b), 'Some psychological aspects of pain', *Amer. J. Psychol.*, vol. 73, p. 80.

PIERCY, M. (1959), 'Testing intellectual impairment', *J. ment. Sci.*, vol. 105, p. 489.

PRIBRAM, K. H. (1968), 'The primate frontal cortex', in A. R. Luria and K. H. Pribram (eds.), *Frontal Lobes and the Regulation of Behavior*, Academic Press.

PRIBRAM, K. H. (1969), 'The neurophysiology of remembering', *Scient. Amer.*, vol. 220, p. 73.

PRIBRAM, K. H., and TUBBS, W. E. (1967), 'The primate frontal cortex', *Science*, vol. 156, p. 1765.

RIBOT, T. (1885), *Diseases of Memory*, Kegan Paul.

ROCHFORD, G. (1969), The breakdown of language associated with organic brain damage, *Thesis offered for D. Phil. Oxon.*

ROCHFORD, G., and WILLIAMS, M. (1962), 'Studies in the development and breakdown of the use of names. I and II', *J. Neurol. Neurosurg. Psychiat.*, vol. 25, pp. 222, 229.

ROCHFORD, G., and WILLIAMS, M. (1963), 'Studies in the development and breakdown of the use of names. III', *J. Neurol. Neurosurg. Psychiat.*, vol. 26, p. 377.

ROCHFORD, G., and WILLIAMS, M. (1964), 'The measurement of language disorders', *Speech Pathol. Ther.*, vol. 7, p. 3.

ROCHFORD, G., and WILLIAMS, M. (1965), 'Studies in the

development and breakdown of the use of names. IV', *J. Neurol. Neurosurg. Psychiat.*, vol. 28, p. 407.

ROMMETVEIT, R., TOCH, H., and SVENDSEN, D. (1969), 'A study of stereoscopic rivalry', *Scand. J. Psychol.*, vol. 9, p. 138.

RUSSELL, W. R. (1959), *Brain, Memory and Learning*, Clarendon Press.

RUSSELL, W. R., and ESPIR, M. L. E. (1961), *Traumatic Aphasia*, Oxford University Press.

RYLANDER, G. (1939), *Personality Changes after Operations on the Frontal Lobes*, Oxford University Press.

SCHILDER, P. (1950), *The Image and Appearance of the Human Body*, International Universities Press.

SEMMES, J. (1968), 'Hemispheric specialization', *Neuropsychol.*, vol. 6, p. 11.

SEMMES, J., WEINSTEIN, S., GHENT, L., and TEUBER, H. L. (1963), 'Correlates of impaired orientation', *Brain*, vol. 86, p. 747.

SERAFETINIDES, E. A., and FALCONER, M. A. (1963), 'Speech disturbances in temporal lobe seizures', *Brain*, vol. 86, p. 333.

SHANKWEILER, D. (1966), 'Dichotically presented melodies', *J. comp. physiol. Psychol.*, vol. 62, p. 115.

SHANKWEILER, D., and HARRIS, K. S. (1966), 'Articulation in aphasia', *Cortex*, vol. 2, p. 277.

SHANKWEILER, D., and STUDDERT-KENNEDY, M. (1959), 'Speech sounds in interaural competition', *Quart. J. exp. Psychol.*, vol. 19, p. 59.

SHERWIN, I. (1966), 'Seizures precipitated by the use of language', *Cortex*, vol. 2, p. 347.

SIMMELL, M. (1956), 'Phantoms in patients with leprosy', *Amer. J. Psychol.*, vol. 69, p. 529.

SIMMELL, M. (1961), 'The absence of phantoms for congenitally missing limbs', *Amer. J. Psychol.*, vol. 74, p. 467.

SIMMELL, M. (1962), 'Phantom experiences following amputation in childhood', *J. Neurol. Neurosurg. Psychiat.*, vol. 25, p. 69.

SIMMELL, M. (1963), 'The psychological after-effects of amputation', *Rehab. Council Bull.*, vol. 6, p. 75.

SMITH, A. (1960), 'Changes in scores of brain-operated schizophrenics', *J. ment. Sci.*, vol. 106, p. 967.

SMITH, A. (1966a), 'Intellectual functions in patients with lateralized frontal tumours', *J. Neurol. Neurosurg. Psychiat.*, vol. 29, p. 52.

SMITH, A. (1966b), 'Speech and other functions after left hemispherectomy', *J. Neurol. Neurosurg. Psychiat.*, vol. 29, p. 467.

SMYTHIES, J. R. (1966), *The Neurological Foundations of Psychiatry*, Blackwell.

SPARKS, R., and GESCHWIND, N. (1968), 'Dichotic listening after section of the neocortical commissures', *Cortex*, vol. 4, p. 3.

SPINNLER, H., and VIGNOLO, L. A. (1966), 'Impaired sound recognition in aphasia', *Cortex*, vol. 2, p. 337.

STEELE-RUSSELL, I., and OCHS, S. (1963), 'Localization and transfer of memory trace', *Brain*, vol. 86, p. 37.

STENGEL, E. (1948), 'Visual alexia and colour agnosia', *J. ment. Sci.*, vol. 94, p. 46.

SYLVESTER, P. E. (1966), 'Parietal lobe deficit in the mentally retarded', *J. Neurol. Neurosurg. Psychiat.*, vol. 29, p. 176.

SYMONDS, C. P. (1937), 'Head injuries', *Proc. Roy. Soc. Med.*, vol. 30, p. 1081.

TALLAND, G. A. (1965), *Deranged Memory*, Academic Press.

THORNDIKE, E. L., and LORGE, I. (1938), *Semantic Word Count* (unpublished).

THORNDIKE, E. L., and LORGE, I. (1944), *The Teacher's Word Book of 30,000 Words*, Bureau of Publications, Teachers College, Columbia University.

TREISMAN, A. (1965), 'Verbal responses and contextual restraints', *J. verb. Learn. verb. Behav.*, vol. 4, p. 118.

TOW, MCD. (1955), *Personality Changes Following Frontal Leucotomy*, Oxford University Press.

VERNON, M. D. (1957), *Backwardness in Reading*, Cambridge University Press.

WALLACE, J. G. (1956), 'Some studies of perception in relation to age', *Brit. J. Psychol.*, vol. 47, p. 283.

WALTER, W. G. (1966), Electrophysiological contributions to psychiatric therapy, *Current Psychological Therapies*, vol. 6, Grune & Stratton.

WALTER, W. G. (1967), 'Electrical signs of association expectancy and decision', *Rec. Adv. Neurol. Physiol.*, suppl. 25.

WARRINGTON, E. K. (1962), 'Completion of visual forms across the hemionopic field', *J. Neurol. Neurosurg. Psychiat.*, vol. 25, p. 208.

WARRINGTON, E. K. (1969), 'Constructional apraxia', in *Handbook of Clinical Neurology*, vol. 4, North-Holland.

WARRINGTON, E. K., and JAMES, M. (1967a), 'Disorders of visual perception with localized cerebral lesions', *Neuropsychol.*, vol. 5, p. 253.

WARRINGTON, E. K., and JAMES, M. (1967b), 'Facial recognition and unilateral cerebral lesions', *Cortex*, vol. 3, p. 317.

WARRINGTON, E. K., and WEISKRANTZ, L. (1968), 'Long-term retention in amnesic patients', *Nature*, vol. 217, p. 972.

WEIGL, E. (1963), 'Deblockierung bildagnostischer Störrungen bei einem aphatiker', *Neuropsychol.*, vol. 1, p. 91.

WEIGL, E. (1964), 'The problem of so-called simultanagnosia', *Neuropsychol.*, vol. 2, p. 189.

WEINSTEIN, E. A., and KELLER, M. J. A. (1963), 'Linguistic patterns of misnaming in brain injury', *Neuropsychol.*, vol. 1, p. 79.

WEINSTEIN, E. A., COLE, M., and MITCHELL, M. S. (1964), 'Agnosia and aphasia', *Arch. Neurol.*, vol. 10, p. 376.

WEINSTEIN, E. A., LYERLEY, O. A., COLE, M. and OZER, M. N. (1966), 'Meaning in jargon aphasia', *Cortex*, vol. 2, p. 166.

WEINSTEIN, S., SERSEN, E. A., and VETTER, R. J. (1964), 'Phantoms in congenital aphasia', *Cortex*, vol. 1, p. 276.

WEINSTEIN, S., SERSEN, E. A., and VETTER, R. J. (1968), 'Phantoms after orchidectomy', *Neuropsychol.*, vol. 6, p. 63.

WEISENBERG, T., and MCBRIDE, K. E. (1935), *Aphasia, A Clinical and Psychological Study*, Oxford University Press.

WEISKRANTZ, L. (1966), 'Experimental studies of amnesia', in C. H. W. Whitty and O. L. Zangwill (eds.), *Amnesia*, Butterworth, ch.1.

WELFORD, A. T. (1958), *Ageing and Human Skill*, Nuffield Foundation.

WERNER, N. (1956), 'Microgenesis and aphasia', *J. abnorm. soc. Psychol.*, vol. 52, p. 347.

WHITTY, C. W. M. (1964), 'Cortical dysarthria', *J. Neurol. Neurosurg. Psychiat.*, vol. 27, p. 507.

WHITTY, C. W. M., and LISHMAN, W. A. (1966), 'Amnesia in cerebral disease', in C. W. M. Whitty and O. L. Zangwill (eds.), *Amnesia*, Butterworth, ch. 2.

WILLIAMS, M. (1950), 'Memory studies with ECT. I and II', *J. Neurol. Neurosurg. Psychiat.*, vol. 13, pp. 30, 314.

WILLIAMS, M. (1952), 'A case of displaced affect following ECT', *Brit. J. med. Psychol.*, vol. 25, p. 156.

WILLIAMS, M. (1954), Memory defects associated with cerebral lesions, *Thesis submitted for D. Phil. Oxon.*

WILLIAMS, M. (1960), 'The effects of past experience in the elderly', *J. ment. Sci.*, vol. 104, p. 783.

WILLIAMS, M. (1965), *Mental Testing in Clinical Practice*, Pergamon.

WILLIAMS, M. (1968), 'The measurement of memory in clinical practice', *Brit. J. soc. clin. Psychol.*, vol. 7, p. 19.

WILLIAMS, M. (1969), 'The psychological assessment of geriatric patients', in P. Mittler (ed.), *The Psychological Assessment of Mental and Physical Handicaps*, Methuen, ch. 11.

WILLIAMS, M., and PENNYBACKER, J. (1954), 'Memory defects in tumours of the third ventricle', *J. Neurol. Neurosurg. Psychiat.*, vol. 17, p. 115.

WILLIAMS, M., and SMITH, H. V. (1954), 'Memory defects in tuberculous meningitis', *J. Neurol. Neurosurg. Psychiat.*, vol. 17, p. 173.

WILLIAMS, M., and ZANGWILL, O. L. (1952), 'Retrograde memory disturbances', *J. Neurol. Neurosurg. Psychiat.*, vol. 15, p. 54.

WOLPERT, I. (1924), 'Simultanagnosia', *Z. Gez. Neurol. Psychiat.*, vol. 93, p. 397.

ZANGWILL, O. L. (1950), 'Amnesia and the generic image', *Quart. J. exp. Psychol.*, vol. 2, p. 7.

ZANGWILL, O. L. (1963), 'The cerebral localization of cerebral function', *Advance Sci.*, vol. 20, p. 1.

ZANGWILL, O. L. (1966), 'The amnesic syndrome', in C. W. M. Whitty and O. L. Zangwill (eds.), *Amnesia*, Butterworth, ch. 3.

ZANGWILL, O. L. (1967), 'The Grünthal-Störrung case of amnesia syndrome', *Brit. J. Psychiat.*, vol. 113, p. 113.

ZINKIN, S., and MILLER, A. J. (1967), 'Memory disturbances after ECS', *Science*, vol. 155, p. 102.

Index

Index

Abercrombie, M. L. J., 66, 156
Acalculia, 75, 80, 121, 122, 123
Affect, 142
Aggression, 25
Agnosia, 58–73
  colour, 60, 75
  finger, 75, 76, 79, 80
  mechanisms in, 69–74
  metaphorphopsia, 59
  object, 59
  prospognosia, 59
  simultanagnosia, 61
  visual inattention, 63
  visual perseveration in, 64
  visual scanning in, 66, 67
  visuo-spatial, 65, 97
  agraphia, 75, 80
  see also Dysgraphia
Akinetic mutism, 18
Alajouanine, T., 110, 156
Allison, R. S., 131, 156
Alexia
  see Dyslexia
Amnesia, 16–24, 33–57
  in childhood, 50
  in ECT, 29, 36, 45
  in head injuries, 35, 41–4
  in Korsakov states, 34–5
  in TBM, 21, 44
  neuropathology of, 52–6
  perception in, 46
  retrograde
  see Retrograde amnesia
Amusia, 82, 84
Amygdaloid nucleus, 30, 32, 54, 99, 138
Anosognosia, 75, 79, 80, 81, 107
Anton's syndrome, 65
Aphasia, 79, 82
  see also Dysphasia
Apraxia, 79, 93–8
  constructional, 95–7
  dressing, 95
  ideational, 94, 95
  ideomotor, 94, 95
  in dementia, 129
  mechanisms, 97, 98
  verbal, 109, 110
Archibald, Y. M., 113, 156
Articulation, 109
Ataxia, 93
Auditory cortex, 90
Auditory pathways, 90
Auditory perception, 82–4

Babcock Test, 39, 126
Bateson, G., 146, 156
Bay, 59, 66
Belmont, I., 63, 68, 92, 156
Bender, M. B., 83, 156
Bender–Gestalt Test, 128
Benton, A., 139, 156

Benton's designs from Memory
  Test, 127
Birch, H. G., 63, 68, 92, 156
Birley, J. L. T., 145, 156
Blakemore, C. D., 114, 156
Body-image disorders, 74–82
Bogan, J. E., 98, 158
Boldrey, E., 78, 161
Boller, F., 84, 85, 156
Brain-stem, 18, 25
  in consciousness, 25, 32
  in memory, 57
Brickner, R. M., 141, 156
Brierley, J. B., 52, 53, 156
Broca's area, 112, 113
Bromley, D. B., 156
Browne, M. W., 158

Cairns, H., 18, 25, 26, 156
Catastrophic reaction, 132
Caudate nucleus, 135
Chapman, J., 23, 160
Chunking
  after frontal lobotomy, 140
  in comprehension, 87
Cingulate gyrus, 53, 54, 135,
  150
Cingulectomy, 135, 143, 144,
  148
Clardy, E. R., 25, 157
Cobb, S., 147, 157
Cognitive dissonance, 146, 147
Cole, M., 79, 80, 164
Concreteness, 131, 132, 135
Conrad, R., 121, 157
Consciousness, 15–27
  in head injury, 17
  in intracranial tumours, 18
  in TBM, 21
  in toxic-infective states, 20
  mechanisms, 23–7

Cooper, R., 144, 157
Cordeau, J. P., 55, 157
Corpus collosum, 26, 98, 99, 115
Costello, C. G., 146, 157
Coxon, M. W., 28, 159
Critchley, M., 59, 60, 61, 64,
  65, 66, 70, 75, 76, 77, 80,
  81, 96, 157
Crow, H. J., 144, 157
Curry, F. K. W., 80, 157

Davison, K., 158
Dementia, 95, 119
  in old age, 124–6
  in focal lesions, 126–33
  mechanisms, 133–40
Depression, 27–32, 126
  in organic states, 25
  in pre-frontal leucotomy, 143
de Renzi, E., 60, 84, 95, 157
Diamond, S. P., 83, 156
Dichotic listening, 87, 88, 89,
  111
Diencephalon, 25, 26, 52, 57
Disorientation, right-left, 80
Duisberg, R. E. H., 158
Dysarthria, 109, 111
Dysgraphia, 101, 116, 117–21
  mechanisms, 121–3
Dyslexia, 101, 116, 117,
  121-3
Dysphasia
  comprehensive, 82–91, 101
  expressive, 99–116
    frequency in, 102
    handedness in, 114–16
    in childhood, 110
    in psychosis, 100–102, 108
    jargon, 105–9
    physical basis of, 112–16
    recovery of, 114

relation to normal speech,
110–12
standard dysphasia, 100–105,
110–12
subcortical areas in, 115
Dysprosody, 109

ECT
effect on depression, 29
effect on memory, 36–8
effect on speech, 110
EEG, 16
in over-arousal, 23, 27
in pre-frontal leucotomy, 140,
148, 149
Efron, R., 89, 157
Eisenson's Test for Dysphasia,
127
Encephalitis lethargica, 20, 24,
25
Epilepsy, 21, 22
petit mal, 19
Ervin, F. R., 22, 157
Espir, M. L. E., 114, 162
Ettlinger, G., 68, 69, 157
Eysenck, H. J., 144, 157

Faglioni, P., 60, 157
Falconer, M. A., 113, 114, 156
Fedio, P., 115, 160
Festinger, L., 146, 157
Filtering, in comprehension, 87
Finger agnosia
see Agnosia
Fornix, 26, 53, 54
Frequency, effect in speech,
102
Freud, S., 107, 157
Friedman, A. M., 21, 157
Frontal leucotomy
effect on intelligence, 134–40

effect on personality, 141–7
effect on physiology, 147–50
Frontal lobes, 70
functions of, 139, 140, 147–50
in comprehension, 113, 120,
122
in dementia, 134–40
scanning defects in, 67
thalamic connexions of, 138
Frost, I., 29, 159
Fulton, J., 155, 157

Gazzaniga, M. S., 55, 89, 98,
114, 157, 158
Gerstmann, J., 75, 158
Gerstmann's syndrome, 75, 80,
81, 119, 122
Gelder, M. G., 145, 160
Geschwind, N., 89, 98, 110,
158, 159
Ghent-Braine, L., 67, 158, 162
Gibbs, F. A., 158
Gloning, I., 59, 60, 61, 65, 67,
71, 81, 122, 158
Gloning, K., 59, 60, 61, 65, 67,
71, 81, 122, 158
Goldstein, K., 131, 132, 158
Goldstein–Scheerer Test, 132,
133
Goodglass, H., 94, 158
Gordon, N., 86, 158
Green, J. R., 146, 158
Greenblatt, M., 147, 158

Haley, J., 156
Halliday, A. M., 30, 37, 158
Halnan, C. R. E., 80, 158
Harb, G., 67, 158
Harris, K. S., 88, 162
Head, H., 101, 154, 158

Herbeg, J., 26, 159
Heschl's gyrus, 90, 91, 99
Hill, B. C., 25, 157
Hippocampus (including hippocampal formation and hippocampal gyrus), 52, 54, 99
Hoff, H., 59, 60, 61, 65, 67, 71, 81, 122, 158
Howes, D. H., 110, 159
Humphrey, M. E., 68, 71, 159
Hurvitz, L. J., 131, 156
Hutt, C., 23, 26, 28, 159
Hutt, J. T., 26, 28, 159
Hypothalamus, 26, 30, 31

Ingram, 86
Intelligence, 125–40

Jackson, D. D., 156
Jackson, J. H., 107, 113, 159
Jambor, K., 80, 159
James, M., 60, 71, 163

Kaplan, E., 94, 158
Kaplan, H. I., 21, 157
Karp, E., 63, 92, 156
Karpor, B. A., 67, 137, 160
Keller, M. J. A., 100, 164
Kelly, D. H. W., 150, 159
Kimura, D., 72, 88, 159
Kinsbourne, M., 63, 65, 68, 107, 109, 116, 159
Korsakov states, 33, 53
Kreeger, L. C., 158

Lancaster, N. P., 29, 159
Lashley, K. S., 55, 159
Lateral ventricle, 54
Lawson, J. S., 23, 160

Lee, D., 159
Leucotomy
  see Frontal leucotomy
Levison, F., 144, 160
Lewin, W. W., 143, 160
L'Hermitte, F., 77, 110, 156
Limbic system, 25, 26, 53, 140, 149
Lishman, W. A., 164
Lorge, I., 102, 103, 163
Luria, A. R., 67, 92, 137, 160
Lyerley, O. A., 164

Magoun, H. W., 25
Mahert, H., 55, 157
Mammillary bodies, 26, 52, 54
Mammillothalmic tract, 54
Marks, I. M., 145, 160
Marshall, J. C., 89, 117, 160
Mayer Gross, W., 20, 45, 132, 160
McBride, K. E., 101, 164
McFie, J., 65, 70, 71, 160
McGhie, A., 23, 160
McGrath, W. B., 158
McKinney, J. P., 72, 160
Medulla, 18
Memory
  in old age, 125
    see also Amnesia
Meyer, V., 144, 160
Microgenesis, theory of, 151
Mid-brain, 25, 26
Miles, T. R., 121, 160
Miller, A. J., 46, 165
Milner, B., 34, 35, 38, 41, 54, 84, 88, 160
Mishkin, M., 139, 160
Mitchell, M. S., 79, 80, 164
Mitchell, S. W., 77, 160

Narcolepsy, 16
Newcombe, F., 89, 117, 160

Occipital lobe, 69, 70, 71, 73
  in body-image, 80–82
  in comprehension, 91–2
Ochs, S., 31, 161
Ojemann, G. A., 115, 160
Oldfield, R. C., 111, 161
Olds, J., 31, 161
Optic pathways, 73
Orbach, J., 67, 161
Orbital leucotomy
  see Frontal leucotomy
Oswald, I., 25, 161
Ottoson, J. O., 30, 161
Ounsted, C., 159
Ozer, M. N., 164

Papez, circuit of, 53
Parietal lobe, 70, 113
  in apraxia, 97
  in body-image disorders, 74,
    80–82
  in comprehension, 86, 113
  in expression, 115
  in reading and writing, 119,
    120, 122
  in vision, 69, 71
Partridge, M., 134, 135, 136,
    138, 140, 141, 161
Penfield, W., 78, 90, 92, 161
Pennybacker, J., 34, 164
Perot, P., 90, 161
Perseveration
  in comprehension loss, 113
  in dementia, 128, 130, 131
  in frontal-lobe deficit, 135, 139
  in jargon aphasia, 108
  in writing, 118
Personality, 140–50

Petrie, A., 143, 144, 147, 148,
    161
Phantom limbs, 76–9
  in children, 78
  supernumerary, 76
Phillips, D. G., 144, 157
Pieczuro, A., 95, 157
Piercy, M. F., 65, 70, 71, 126,
    160, 161
Pierre-Marie Test, 84
Pineal body, 26
Pituitary gland, 26
Pons, 18, 26
Porteus Maze Test, 136
Pribram, K. H., 56, 138, 139,
    160, 161
Prosopagnosia, 59
Pulvinar, 115

Quatember, R., 60, 158

Reticular formation, 25, 26
Retrograde amnesia, 41–50
  after ECT 45, 46
  after head injury, 41–4
  after TBM, 44
  compared to normal
    forgetting, 46–50
  shrinkage, 41
Rey Davis Test, 37
Ribot, T., 41, 161
Rochford, G., 99, 101, 102,
    103, 104, 107, 109, 111, 117,
    131, 161
Rommetveit, T., 63
Roth, M., 20, 132, 160
Russell, W. R., 15, 17, 41, 50,
    114, 162
Rutherford, D. R., 90, 157
Rylander, G., 141, 162

Sargeant, W., 150, 159
Scanning
  in backward readers, 119
  in dyslexia, 121
  in left-handedness, 67
  in visual agnosia, 66, 67
Scheerer, M., 131, 132, 158
Schilder, P., 79, 162
Schizophrenia
  EEG in, 149
  effect of pre-frontal leucotomy
    on, 143
  speech disorders in, 100, 108,
    120
Scoville, 34, 54
Seashore Test, 84, 88
Semantic frequency, 103
Semmes, J., 72, 81, 162
Senility, speech disorders in,
  100, 101, 102, 120
Serafetinides, E. A., 113, 162
Sersen, E. A., 78, 164
Shankweiler, D., 88, 89, 162
Sherwin, I., 22, 162
Simmel, M., 77, 78, 162
Simultanagnosia, 61
Slater, E., 20, 132, 160
Sleep, 20, 22, 25
Smith, A., 112, 139, 162
Smith, H. V., 15, 21, 34, 39,
  45, 164
Smythies, J. R., 57, 163
Solomon, H. C., 147, 158
Sparks, R., 89, 163
Sperry, R. W., 55, 89, 98, 114,
  157, 163
Spinnler, H., 60, 82, 157, 163
Split-brain preparations, 55, 89
Stedman, H. F., 158
Steele-Russell, I., 55, 163
Steinert, R. R., 29, 159

Stengel, E., 60, 61, 163
Studdert-Kennedy, M., 89,
  162
Svendsen, D., 63, 162
Sylvester, P. E., 139, 163
Symonds, C. P., 41, 163

Talland, G. A., 34, 35, 38, 41,
  163
Taylor, J. G., 86, 158
Taylor, M., 156
TBM
  see Tuberculous meningitis
Temporal lobe, 54, 70, 88
  frontal connexions, 138
  in reading and writing, 122
  in speech, 112–16, 120
Temporal lobectomy,
  effect on comprehension,
    88–92
  effect on memory, 34
  effect on perseveration, 144,
    146
Terman Merrill Test, 106
Teuber, H. H., 162
Thalamus, 25, 26, 52, 54, 99,
  115
Third ventricle, 18, 54, 99
Thorndike, E. L., 102, 103,
  163
Toch, H., 63, 162
Tow, McD., 136, 138, 163
Transitional probabilities, 86,
  87
Treisman, A., 87, 163
Tubbs, W. E., 139, 140, 161
Tuberculous meningitis
  (TBM), 15, 20, 21, 39
Tschabitscher, H., 158

Uncus, 54

Ventricle
 see Third ventricle and
  Lateral ventricle
Vernon, M. D., 119, 163
Vetter, R. J., 78, 164
Vigilance, 23
Vignolo, L. A., 82, 84, 85, 95,
  156, 157, 163
Visual disorders
 see Agnosia
Visual imagery, 68, 119
Visual pathways, 73

WAIS, 96, 124, 126, 134
Wakefulness, 15
 see also Sleep
Wallace, J. G., 68, 163
Walter, C. J. S., 150, 159
Walter, W. G., 145, 148, 163
Warrington, E. K., 38, 60, 63,
  65, 66, 68, 71, 72, 96, 97,
  102, 107, 109, 117, 159, 163
Weakland, J., 156
Wechler Memory Test, 127
Welford, A. T., 124, 164
Weigl, E., 61, 104, 163, 164
Weigl–Goldstein–Scheerer
  Test, 131, 133, 134
Weinstein, E. A., 79, 80, 86,
  100, 107, 109, 164

Weinstein, S., 78, 162, 164
Weisenberg, T., 101, 164
Weiskrantz, L., 38, 45, 46, 163,
  164
Wepman, J. M., 113, 156
Werner, N., 151, 164
Whitty, C. W. M., 33, 110,
  164
Wick, W. S., 158
Williams, M., 15, 17, 21, 34,
  36, 37, 38, 39, 41, 45, 80,
  103, 104, 111, 117, 125, 126,
  133, 134, 161, 164, 165
Wingfield, A., 111, 161
Wolpert, I., 61, 165
Word association, in jargon
  aphasia, 109
Word blindness, 119, 121, 122
Word deafness, 82, 84–91
 in children, 85, 86
 in jargon aphasia, 86
 mechanisms, 86–91
Wright, G. H., 80, 158
Wyke, M., 68, 157

Yarhuss, A. L., 67, 137, 160

Zangwill, O. L., 34, 41, 46, 65,
  68, 70, 71, 114, 159, 160,
  165
Zinkin, S., 46, 165